Pharmacology – Research, Safety Testing and Regulation

The Pharmacological Guide to Sofosbuvir

PHARMACOLOGY – RESEARCH, SAFETY TESTING AND REGULATION

Additional books and e-books in this series can be found on Nova's website under the Series tab.

PHARMACOLOGY – RESEARCH, SAFETY TESTING AND REGULATION

THE PHARMACOLOGICAL GUIDE TO SOFOSBUVIR

VIJAY GAYAM
EDITOR

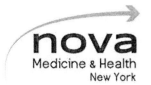

Copyright © 2019 by Nova Science Publishers, Inc.

All rights reserved. No part of this book may be reproduced, stored in a retrieval system or transmitted in any form or by any means: electronic, electrostatic, magnetic, tape, mechanical photocopying, recording or otherwise without the written permission of the Publisher.

We have partnered with Copyright Clearance Center to make it easy for you to obtain permissions to reuse content from this publication. Simply navigate to this publication's page on Nova's website and locate the "Get Permission" button below the title description. This button is linked directly to the title's permission page on copyright.com. Alternatively, you can visit copyright.com and search by title, ISBN, or ISSN.

For further questions about using the service on copyright.com, please contact:
Copyright Clearance Center
Phone: +1-(978) 750-8400   Fax: +1-(978) 750-4470   E-mail: info@copyright.com.

NOTICE TO THE READER

The Publisher has taken reasonable care in the preparation of this book, but makes no expressed or implied warranty of any kind and assumes no responsibility for any errors or omissions. No liability is assumed for incidental or consequential damages in connection with or arising out of information contained in this book. The Publisher shall not be liable for any special, consequential, or exemplary damages resulting, in whole or in part, from the readers' use of, or reliance upon, this material. Any parts of this book based on government reports are so indicated and copyright is claimed for those parts to the extent applicable to compilations of such works.

Independent verification should be sought for any data, advice or recommendations contained in this book. In addition, no responsibility is assumed by the Publisher for any injury and/or damage to persons or property arising from any methods, products, instructions, ideas or otherwise contained in this publication.

This publication is designed to provide accurate and authoritative information with regard to the subject matter covered herein. It is sold with the clear understanding that the Publisher is not engaged in rendering legal or any other professional services. If legal or any other expert assistance is required, the services of a competent person should be sought. FROM A DECLARATION OF PARTICIPANTS JOINTLY ADOPTED BY A COMMITTEE OF THE AMERICAN BAR ASSOCIATION AND A COMMITTEE OF PUBLISHERS.

Additional color graphics may be available in the e-book version of this book.

Library of Congress Cataloging-in-Publication Data

ISBN: 978-1-53616-476-3
Library of Congress Control Number:2019950994

Published by Nova Science Publishers, Inc. † New York

Chapter 4	Management of HCV Infection with Sofosbuvir-Based Regimens in Patients with Medical Co-Morbidities *Amrendra Kumar Mandal, Venu Madhav Konala, Sreedhar Adapa, Srikanth Naramala, Benjamin Tiongson, and Vijay Gayam*	91
Chapter 5	Management of Patients Co-Infected with HCV/HIV and HCV/HBV *Amrendra Kumar Mandal, Jasdeep Singh Sidhu, Benjamin Tiongson, Pavani Garlapati, Pallav Patel and Vijay Gayam*	113
Chapter 6	Sofosbuvir Treatment of Hepatitis C in People with Psychiatric Illness and Substance Use Disorders *Benjamin Tiongson, Oluwole Jegede, Olaniyi Olayinka, Pavani Garlapati, Amrendra Kumar Mandal, Vijay Gayam and Jason Hershberger*	133
Chapter 7	Sofosbuvir and Chronic Hepatitis C Treatment Failure *Arshpal Gill, Priya Batta, Amrendra Kumar Mandal, Pavani Garlapati, Vijay Gayam and Smruti Mohanty*	171

Editor's Contact Information   187

Index   189

Related Nova Publications   197

CONTENTS

Preface vii

Chapter 1 Pharmacological Principles of Sofosbuvir 1
*Ramakanth Pata, Pavani Garlapati,
Venu Madhav Konala, Sreedhar Adapa,
Srikanth Naramala and Vijay Gayam*

Chapter 2 Sofosbuvir in Non-Cirrhotic Patients
with Chronic Hepatitis C Infection 39
*Amrendra Kumar Mandal, Benjamin Tiongson,
Eric O. Then, Vijay Gayam and Vinaya Gaduputi*

Chapter 3 Initial Management Options Involving
Sofosbuvir in Chronic Hepatitis C Infection
with Liver Cirrhosis 59
*Vijay Gayam, Arshpal Gill, Ricky Lali,
Pavani Garlapati, Eric O. Then,
Srikanth Maddika, and Vinaya Gaduputi*

PREFACE

The Pharmacological Guide to Sofosbuvir comprises of 7 comprehensive chapters on the pharmacology, safety, efficacy, and tolerability of Sofosbuvir in the treatment of chronic hepatitis C infection (CHC).

The discovery of direct-acting antiretroviral drugs has revolutionized the treatment of CHC. In Chapter 1, Dr. Pata et al. focuses on Sofosbuvir, which acts by inhibiting NS5B polymerase of the HCV virus, thereby inhibiting the replication of the virus. It is an exhaustive discussion of Sofosbuvir and its pharmacological saga.

Sofosbuvir has been utilized as the backbone in a variety of combination regimens for the treatment of CHC. In Chapter 2, Dr. Mandal et al. reviewed the use of Sofosbuvir in Non-cirrhotic Patients with Chronic Hepatitis C Infection. In Chapter 3, the authors reviewed the initial management options involving Sofosbuvir in Chronic Hepatitis C Infection with Liver Cirrhosis.

The treatment of chronic hepatitis C in a patient with medical co-morbidities brings certain challenges. One should take into account changes in drug metabolism in patients with renal impairment or decompensated liver cirrhosis; also drug-drug interactions in transplanted patients should be considered. In Chapter 4, Dr. Mandal et al. reviewed the management of HCV infection with Sofosbuvir-based regimens in patients with medical co-morbidities.

Hepatitis B, Hepatitis C and, Human immunodeficiency viruses share similar routes of transmission, the likelihood of increased morbidity and mortality for the number of complications arising from these conditions remain significant. Furthermore, co-infection leads to serious livers problems arising from more aggressive liver disease, advancing fibrosis, and earlier progression to end-stage liver disease. In Chapter 5, Dr. Mandal et al. reviewed the management of patients co-infected with HCV/HIV and HCV/HBV.

There is a high comorbidity of chronic Hepatitis C among individuals with mental illness, particularly among the subpopulation of people who use drugs. In Chapter 6, Dr. Tiongson et al. reviewed the Sofosbuvir treatment of Hepatitis C in People with Psychiatric Illness and Substance Use Disorders. In Chapter 7, Dr. Gill et al. discussed the factors associated with direct-acting antiviral (DAA) failure, including Cirrhosis, Vitamin D deficiency, Renal Failure, and Co-Infection with HIV. The impact and role of viral resistance variants in HCV, as well as the management of DAA failure using Sofosbuvir-based regimens, were also reviewed.

I am very thankful to all the authors for their outstanding contributions. I would also like to appreciate the efforts of the dedicated team of Nova Science Publishers, Inc.

Dr. Vijay Gayam, MD
Editor

In: The Pharmacological Guide to Sofosbuvir   ISBN: 978-1-53616-476-3
Editor: Vijay Gayam   © 2019 Nova Science Publishers, Inc.

Chapter 1

PHARMACOLOGICAL PRINCIPLES OF SOFOSBUVIR

Ramakanth Pata[1,*], *MD, Pavani Garlapati*[1,†], *MD, Venu Madhav Konala*[2,‡], *MD, Sreedhar Adapa*[3,§], *MD, Srikanth Naramala*[4,ǁ], *MD and Vijay Gayam*[5,#], *MD*

[1]Department of Internal Medicine, Interfaith Medical Center, Brooklyn, NY, US
[2]Department of Internal Medicine, Divison of Medical Oncology, Ashland Bellefonte Cancer Center, Ashland, KY, US
[3]Division of Nephrology, The Nephrology Group, CA, US
[4]Department of Internal Medicine, Division of Rheumatology, Adventist Medical Center, Hanford, CA, US
[6]Department of Internal Medicine, Interfaith Medical Center, Brooklyn, NY, US

---

* Corresponding Author's E-mail: cookybrey1@gmail.com.
† Author's E-mail: docpavanireddy@gmail.com.
‡ Author's E-mail: drvenumadhav@gmail.com.
§ Author's E-mail: sreedharadapa@gmail.com.
ǁ Author's E-mail: dr.srikanth83@gmail.com.
Author's E-mail: vgayam@interfaithmedical.org.

Abstract

Hepatitis C virus (HCV), a member of the Flaviviridae family, is the leading cause of morbidity and mortality related to liver failure. It has surpassed alcoholism as the most common cause of liver transplantation. The estimated global prevalence of HCV is around 2.5% of the population (177.5 million). It is also believed that this estimate is only conservative and many go undetected. HCV is known to cause acute and chronic hepatitis with cirrhosis and hepatocellular carcinoma as complications. Also, many extrahepatic diseases are also associated with HCV. Screening high-risk individuals not only is cost-effective but also prevents morbidity related to its consequences. Treatment of HCV has significantly evolved, with research focusing on drugs that are more effective with higher cure rates and shorter duration of therapy. Earlier therapies involved interferon and ribavirin, which were associated with longer courses of treatment and more adverse effects. The discovery of direct-acting antiretroviral drugs has revolutionized the treatment of HCV. Research is still ongoing to discover a drug with even finer attributes. The following is a chapter that focuses on Sofosbuvir, which is one example of direct-acting antiviral drugs. Sofosbuvir acts by inhibiting NS5B polymerase of the HCV virus, thereby inhibiting the replication of the virus. As the gene encoding for this enzyme is conserved in all genotypes of HCV (Types 1-7), therefore making it one of the choices in any HCV genotype-related infection. Sofosbuvir is also one of the drugs that are favored in a unique population; may it be pediatrics or geriatrics or even liver transplant recipients. Furthermore, the side effects and pharmacokinetic profile makes it an exciting choice as one of the components of the direct-acting antiviral regimen. The following is an exhaustive discussion of Sofosbuvir and its pharmacological saga.

Keywords: Sofosbuvir, HCV genotypes, NS5B inhibitors, NS3/4A protease inhibitors, NS5A inhibitors, pharmacokinetics, mechanism of action, dosing regimens, contraindications, adverse effects, P-glycoprotein, BCRP, drug-drug interactions, resistance

ABBREVIATIONS

DAA	Direct-acting antiviral agents
HCV	Hepatitis C virus
HIV	Human Immunodeficiency Virus
HBV	Hepatitis B virus
SVR	Sustained viral response

1. INTRODUCTION AND HISTORY

Hepatitis C virus (HCV), a member of the Flaviviridae family, with its dexterous glycoprotein envelop encasing single-strand RNA, and a burgeoning accouterment is currently considered the leading cause of liver transplantation. It is estimated that around 2.4 million people in the United States are infected with hepatitis C virus accounting for a significant proportion of patients with liver disease. Prevalence of HCV infection is higher in certain groups viz Baby boomers and illicit drug users. People born between 1945- 1965, referred to as Baby Boomers are five times more likely to have HCV, probably related to the transmission patterns before the adoption of Infection control protocols. Center for Disease Control and Prevention (CDC) recommends the" baby boomers" be offered HCV screening test. As the primary route of transmission being bodily fluids including blood, screening should be offered for high-risk personnel, including Intravenous drug users and recipient of donated blood products and organs before 1992. Not just the prevalence of HCV infection is alarming, but it can leave a catastrophic clinical footprint [1].

The clinical sequel of HCV infection can result in a spectrum of manifestations ranging from transient acute Hepatitis to a chronic Hepatitis with a risk of progression to cirrhosis. Among patients with cirrhosis, there is 1-5% annual risk of hepatocellular carcinoma and 3-6% annual risk of hepatic decompensation, for which the risk of death in the following year is 15-20%. The average age of death is as per the estimates is 59 years [1].

Earlier to 2011, the therapies for HCV consisted of Interferon and Ribavirin that required tardy treatment protocols with lower cure rates and adverse side effects. The current era of directly acting antiviral therapies has revolutionized treatment protocols with higher cure rates and abbreviated treatment courses. BY inhibiting various nonstructural proteins, these direct-acting antiviral drugs act on very proliferating machinery of the virus, thereby achieving higher cure rates. Cure rates in HCV are consistent with the absence of detectable virus 12 weeks after completion of treatment, designated as the sustained virological response (SVR12) [2].

One such drug in this direct-acting antiviral regimen is Sofosbuvir. Sofosbuvir acts by inhibiting NS5B polymerase of the HCV virus, the gene encoding for this enzyme is conserved in all genotypes of HCV (Types 1-7), therefore making it one of the choices in any HCV genotype-related infection. Further, the side effects and pharmacokinetic profile makes it an exciting choice as one of the components of the direct-acting antiviral regimen. Sofosbuvir, discovered by Michael Sofia, the launch of which was the fastest of any new drug in the USA. It not only received the FDA's breakthrough designation but also it is on the "World Health Organization's list of essential medicines [3, 4].

2. PHARMACOLOGICAL TARGETS OF HEPATITIS C VIRUS

Hepatitis C virus is a unique virus in that it exhibits remarkable genetic heterogeneity, thus hindering the discovery of a universal vaccine or a universal therapy using the current understanding of the pharmacological principles. A total of seven different genotypes have been identified, and these different genotypes differ at 30-35% of nucleotide sites [5].

Within each genotype, HCV is further classified into subtypes that differ at fewer than 15% of nucleotide sites. Amongst genotypes, transmissibility does not seem to differ, whereas the rate of disease progression and response to treatment with current therapies differ. Even the subtypes exhibit a different response to therapies. HCV subtype 1a tend to have higher relapse rates with certain HCV treatments compared with invidious with subtype 1b. HCV genome consists of a positive sense, single-stranded RNA which encodes three structural proteins (Core, E1, E2), the ion channel protein p7, six nonstructural proteins (NS2, NS3, NS4A, NS4B, NS5A, and NS5 B) [6, 7].

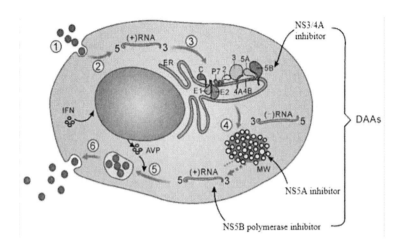

Figure 1a. Image Borrowed from Medical illustrator. David. Cleveland Clinic. This image illustrates the pharmacological targets that act on HCV replication.

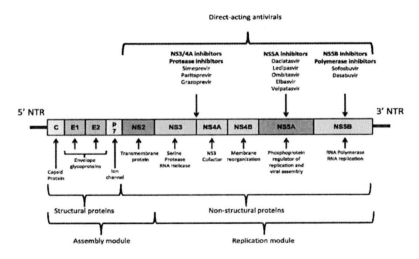

Figure 1b. The figure illustrates various drugs that are currently available in the market and their mechanism of action.

HCV replicates entirely in the cytoplasm. It does not establish latency, and it is curable. Cure of HCV is synonymous with achieving an SVR12, which is defined as no measurable HCV RNA in the blood following cessation of treatment and stands for a sustained virological response. SVR12 is usually assessed 12 weeks following treatment cessation. Achieving SVR12 decreases the progression of liver disease and reduces liver-related and all-cause mortality. On average, almost a trillion HCV particles are produced in an infected individual each day [8].

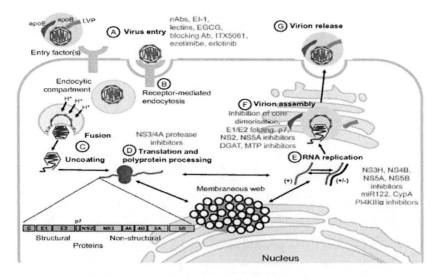

Figure 2. Image borrowed from Gut Journal. There are many investigational drugs currently in research for inhibiting the replication of HCV. These are illustrated in the figure with mechanisms of action.

Earlier regimens consisted of a prolonged regimen of subcutaneously administered IFN-a (or peg IFN-a) with or without Ribavirin which achieved low SVR and had poor tolerability. Currently, several antivirals that directly target various steps in HCV lifecycle so-called DAAs (Direct-acting antivirals) are the mainstay of the therapy. DAAs are administered orally, have few side effects, are taken for a period of anywhere from 8 to 24 weeks, and achieve high cure rates. In certain clinical scenarios, Ribavirin is still used in combination with DAAs to improve SVR12. Interferon treatment is not anymore used as a first or second line.

Available DAAs target three major sites in the HCV life cycle, the NS3 protease, the NS5B polymerase, and NS5A (See Figure 1a and 1b). Some other investigational drugs that can inhibit HCV replication are shown in Figure 2.

2.1. A Brief Overview of the Direct-Acting Antiviral Drugs

2.1.1. NS3 /4A Protease Inhibitors

Inhibition of NS3/4A protease prevents the cleavage of the viral polyprotein and formation of the replication complex. Drugs that inhibit NS3/4A inhibitors include Boceprevir, Telaprevir, Simeprevir, Asunaprevir, Grazoprevir, Voxilaprevir, Telaprevir, and Paritaprevir. These NS3/4A inhibitors are not recommended in patients with current or prior history of decompensated liver disease or with CTP score (Child-Turcotte-Pugh) >6 [9, 10].

2.1.2. NS5B Inhibitors

The NS5B enzyme is essential for HCV replication as it catalyzes the synthesis of the complementary minus-strand RNA and subsequent genomic plus-strand RNA. There are two types of NS5B Rdrp (RNA dependent RNA polymerase) inhibitors - nucleotide and non-nucleoside inhibitors. The nucleotide inhibitors are active site inhibitors (like Sofosbuvir), whereas the non-nucleoside inhibitors are allosteric inhibitors. (Allosteric inhibition: Binding of one ligand decreases the effect of other). Drugs that inhibit NS5B include Sofosbuvir and Dasabuvir. Dasabuvir is an example of Non-nucleoside polymerase inhibitor [11-14].

2.1.3. NS5A Inhibitors

NS5A encodes a protein essential to replication machinery of HCV and is critical in the assembly of new infectious viral particles. Drugs that inhibit NS5A include Ombitasvir, Ledipasvir, Daclatasvir, Elbasvir, and Velpatasvir [15, 16].

Resistance to these drugs has been described. The HCV undergoes amino acid substitutions called polymorphisms that render the virus resistant to the effect of these drugs. These viral variants are termed "Resistant associated Substitutions." Presently the most clinically significant RASs are in the NS5A position for genotypes 1a and 3. The HCV NS5B polymerase enzyme lacks a proofreading function and has poor fidelity, thus susceptible to numerous mutations leading to so-called Resistance-associated Variants (RAVs). Fortunately, nucleotide NS5B polymerase inhibitors have a high genetic barrier to resistance; almost three or more RAVs are required for a full resistance.

In contrast, Non-nucleoside NS5B inhibitors, NS3/4A protease inhibitors, and NS5A inhibitors have a low genetic barrier to resistance, meaning that only one or two amino acid substitutions result in lack of drug efficacy. Compounding the clinical impact of NS5A RASs is their ability to maintain high replication competence (aka Relative fitness) in the absence of continued drug pressure, allowing them to remain dominant viral quasi-species for prolonged periods (years) relative to NS3/4A protease or NS5B nucleotide polymerase inhibitor RASs, which are typically less fit and tend to disappear over several months, being overcome by more fit wild type virus species. Thus to prevent the emergence of drug resistance, monotherapy should be avoided, and hence, HCV treatment always requires a combination. It is therefore prudent to also consider combination therapy for Sofosbuvir, though there is a high genetic barrier to resistance [17].

3. PHARMACOLOGY OF SOFOSBUVIR

3.1. The Unique Chemistry of Sofosbuvir

Many nucleoside analogs that have been examined before the entry of Sofosbuvir into the market exhibited relatively low potency, probably due to the slow enzymatic addition of first of the Phosphate groups, to form active Triphosphate form. To obviate this slow phosphorylation, ProTide design was incorporated into Sofosbuvir. The ProTide technology is a prodrug approach designed to deliver nucleotide analog (as monophosphate) into the cell, which is already mono phosphorylated. (ProTide: PROdrug + nucleoTIDE). The phosphate group is thus built into the structure of the drug during synthesis. However, the addition of phosphate would restrict the entry of the drug into the cell. Additional groups are attached to the phosphorus to temporarily mask the two negative charges of the phosphate group, thereby facilitating entry of the drug into the infected cell. Thus this ProTide design bypasses slow phosphorylation step, yet enters the cell fast enough without regard to the phosphate group that was attached during drug synthesis to bypass the first phosphorylation step [18].

Thus Sofosbuvir is a prodrug based on uridine analog which is phosphorylated (See Figure 3).

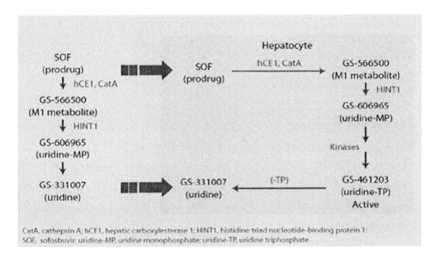

Figure 3. The figure illustrates the steps in the metabolism of Sofosbuvir. Activation, and deactivation.

3.2. Mechanism of Action

Sofosbuvir inhibits the Hepatitis C NS5B protein [36]. The NS5B protein is an RNA-dependent RNA polymerase critical for the viral reproduction cycle. Sofosbuvir is a prodrug. It is metabolized to the active antiviral agent GS-461203 (2'-deoxy-2'-α-fluoro-β-C-methyluridine-5'-triphosphate). GS-461203 serves as a defective substrate for the NS5B protein, which is the viral RNA polymerase, thus acts as an inhibitor of viral RNA synthesis [19].

3.3. Steric Hindrance of Sofosbuvir

Other proposed mechanism of Sofosbuvir is by steric hindrance.

Steric hindrance is the congestion-related brake caused by the physical presence of the surrounding ligands that may slow down or prevent reactions. Although sofosbuvir has a 3' hydroxyl group to act as a nucleophile for an incoming NTP, its nucleotide analog (similar to 2'-deoxy-2'-α-fluoro-β-C-methylcytidine) is proposed to act as a chain terminator due to steric hindrance with the incoming NTP [20].

3.4. Pharmacokinetics

Sofosbuvir is dosed at 400 mg and taken once daily. Sofosbuvir, a prodrug is only administered orally. The peak concentration after oral administration is 0.5–2 hours post-dose, regardless of the initial dose. The half-life of sofosbuvir is 0.4 hours. Bioavailability is 92% in some studies, although the absolute bioavailability is estimated to be around at least 80% based on radiolabeled data [21, 22].

3.4.1. Effect of Food

Relative to fasting conditions, the administration of a single dose of Sofosbuvir with a standardized high fat meal did not substantially affect the maximum concentration (Cmax) or area under the curve (AUC). Although some studies report increased exposure of Sofosbuvir has been demonstrated after a fat meal, this does not translate into an increased likelihood of toxicities because of its high therapeutic index. Therefore, sofosbuvir can be administered without regard to food.

Sofosbuvir exhibits time-independent, near-linear pharmacokinetics across a range of doses. Race and gender did not significantly affect the pharmacokinetics [21, 22].

3.4.2. Activation of the Drug (See Figure 3)

Sofosbuvir is quickly activated to its active triphosphate form GS-461203 occurs in Liver and requires three coordinated steps that include hydrolysis, cleavage, and repeat phosphorylation.

1. Hydrolysis: Hydrolysis of the carboxylate ester is carried out either by of the enzymes cathepsin A (cat A) or carboxylesterase 1(CES1).
2. Cleavage: Hydrolysis is followed by cleaving of the phosphoramidite by the enzyme histidine triad nucleotide-binding protein 1 (HINT1).
3. Repeat Phosphorylation: The cleaved product undergoes repeat phosphorylation yielding the active molecule GS-461203. This phosphorylation occurs through the Pyrimidine nucleotide biosynthetic pathway [22].

3.4.3. Inactivation of the Drug

The drug is inactivated by dephosphorylation to GS-331077, which is the pharmacologically inactive nucleoside and the main circulating metabolite. Peak plasma concentration of this metabolite occurs 2-4 hours postdose. The half-life of GS-331077 is 27 hours. This metabolite cannot be rephosphorylated, lacks anti-viral activity, and exits the cell and excreted via a combination of glomerular filtration and tubular secretion [22, 23].

3.4.4. Protein Binding and Excretion

Plasma protein binding of sofosbuvir is 61–65%, while GS-331077 has minimal binding. Following a single 400 mg oral dose of sofosbuvir, 80%

is excreted in the urine, 14% in feces, and 2.5% in expired air recovery. However, of the urine recovery, 78% was the metabolite (GS-331007), and 3.5% was sofosbuvir [22, 23].

3.4.5. Pharmacokinetics in HIV

Sofosbuvir AUC is 60% higher, and GS-331007 AUC is 39% lower in HIV infected persons compared with HIV negative persons. The mechanism for this is unclear, and the dose need not be modified [23].

4. DOSING CONSIDERATIONS

4.1. Dosing in Hepatic Impairment

Exposure to Sofosbuvir (measured as AUC - Area under Curve) is increased 2.3 fold in moderate hepatic impairment defined as Child-Pugh B. Sofosbuvir AUC is increased 2.5 fold in severe hepatic impairment (Child-Pugh C). However, the AUC of 331007 remains unchanged in moderate or severe hepatic impairment. No dose adjustment is needed for this population, and available data suggest Sofosbuvir is safe and effective in individuals with decompensated cirrhosis when combined with appropriate DAA [24-28].

4.2. Dosing in Renal Impairment

Because the primary route of excretion of the metabolite is via a combination of glomerular filtration and tubular secretion, renal impairment has a significant impact on the pharmacokinetics of Sofosbuvir.

Sofosbuvir and GS-331007 pharmacokinetics are affected by renal impairment [29].

GFR of 50-80 ml/min/1.7 m^2: Sofosbuvir and GS-331007 AUC increased by about 60% in those with GFR 50-80 ml/min/1.7 m^2. No dose adjustment is required GFR of 30-50 ml/min/1.7 m^2: The AUC is increased by two-fold in this population. NO dose adjustment is required, as many studies demonstrated safety and tolerability. GFR < 30 ml/min/1.73 m^2: Sofosbuvir should not be used until more data is available on the safety and appropriate dosing is available, as significant increases in AUC is seen [23].

End stage renal disease (ESRD) requiring dialysis: Sofosbuvir should not be used until more data is available on the safety and appropriate dosing is available, as significant increases in AUC is seen.

In contrast, there is accumulating evidence on safety and efficacy with the use of sofosbuvir-based regimens in those with an eGFR <30 mL/min probably because of its high therapeutic index [30, 31].

For CKD stage 1, 2 and 3, No dosage adjustment is required for regimens that include Sofosbuvir viz. Sofosbuvir (400 mg)/Ledipasvir (90 mg) or Sofosbuvir (400 mg)/Velpatasvir (100 mg) [23].

4.3. Pregnancy and Breastfeeding

Sofosbuvir alone has been assigned a Pregnancy Category B by the FDA (meaning that there are no adequate and well-controlled studies in pregnant women but animal reproduction studies have not demonstrated a risk to the fetus and, or that adverse effects have been seen in animal studies, but adequate and well-controlled studies in pregnant women have not, in any trimester) [32].

However, Ribavirin, a medication that is often given together with Sofosbuvir sometimes, to treat Hepatitis C, is assigned a Pregnancy Category X (contraindicated in pregnancy) by the FDA. Pregnant women with hepatitis C who take ribavirin have shown some cases of congenital disabilities and death in their fetus. It is recommended that Sofosbuvir/Ribarivin combinations be avoided in pregnant females and their male sexual partners to reduce harmful fetal defects caused by ribavirin. Females who could potentially become pregnant should undergo a pregnancy test 2 months before starting the Sofosbuvir/ribavirin/

peginterferon combination treatment, monthly throughout the treatment, and six months post-treatment to reduce the risk of fetal harm in case of accidental pregnancy [33].

It is unknown whether Sofosbuvir and Ribavirin pass into breastmilk; therefore, it is recommended that the mother does not breastfeed during treatment with Sofosbuvir alone or in combination with Ribavirin [32]. If a directly acting anti-viral regimen is chosen, as is currently, often the case, the other components of the combination therapy also should be verified if it is safe in pregnancy. Until further studies are established, Sofosbuvir based regimen are not preferred.

4.4. Sofosbuvir Use in Pediatrics

4.4.1. Age 12 Years and Older

Sofosbuvir with Ledipasvir has been approved by FDA for use in pediatric patients 12 years of age and older or weighing at least 77 pounds (35 kilograms) with HCV genotype 1, 4, 5 or 6 infections without cirrhosis (liver disease) or with mild cirrhosis. The safety, pharmacokinetics, and efficacy of Sofosbuvir with Ledipasvir for the treatment of HCV genotype 1,4,5,6 infection were established in an open-label, multicenter clinical trials [34]. Most common adverse effects include fatigue and headache.

An Egyptian study demonstrated that no adverse cardiovascular events, including bradyarrhythmias, were observed in HCV infected children and adolescents treated with Sofosbuvir/Ledipasvir without any other co-morbidities. Although it must be emphasized that Sofosbuvir must be avoided in patients, including children taking Amiodarone as serious adverse cardiovascular effects have been observed [35].

Sofosbuvir in combination with ribavirin is indicated for the treatment of pediatric patients 12 years of age and older or weighing at least 77 pounds (35 kilograms) with genotype 2 or 3 HCV infection without cirrhosis or with mild cirrhosis. This was evaluated in an open-label clinical trial. The most common adverse effects being fatigue, headache, and nausea [32].

4.4.2. Age 6 to 12 Years

Although not yet approved by the FDA, a study published in Hepatology found the all-oral regimen of Ledipasvir – Sofosbuvir combination to be highly effective and well-tolerated in children 6 to <12 years old. IN this open-label study, Ledipasvir 45mg- sofosbuvir 200 mg ± ribavirin was given to participants administered as two fixed-dose combination tablets 22.5/100 mg once a day for 12 or 24 weeks. Ribavirin was administered with the dose depending on HCV genotype and cirrhosis status. Preliminary data suggest that this combination is safe, effective, and pharmacokinetic profile is similar to adults — the most common adverse effects headache, Pyrexia, and Abdominal Pain. The treatment did not have any significant effects on pubertal development. The conclusion of this study was "A fixed-dose combination of Ledipasvir and Sofosbuvir ± Ribavirin was well tolerated and highly effective for treatment-naïve or interferon-experienced children aged 6 to <12 with chronic HCV genotype 1, 3, and four infections" [36].

It must be remembered that, in choosing a regimen, the same principles for prescribing anti HCV therapy in adults should be extrapolated to children that include the probability of Hep B reactivation in children co-infected with HCV/HBV. FDA categorizes this as a boxed warning even in pediatric patients [34].

4.5. Sofosbuvir in Geriatrics

Rates of Hepatitis C virus are disproportionately high in older patients. Patients born between 1945-1965 represent the highest proportion of about 70% of HCV infected individuals in the USA. Treating elderly patients with Pegylated Interferon and Ribavirin, which was considered as the standard therapy in the last decade, has been challenging due to the frequent presence of multiple co-morbidities like coronary artery disease and diabetes in the elderly and high discontinuation rates caused by adverse events. The availability of non-interferon, direct-acting agents (DAA) represents a major paradigm shift in anti-HCV therapy [37, 38].

Rather many cost-effective studies reported pharmaco-economic advantages of screening and treating HCV infected elderly with Interferon-free therapy using DAA agents while mitigating the health consequences of HCV infection [39, 40]. The interferon-free regimen is preferable for some reasons that include tolerability, adherence, adverse effects like increased risk of hemolytic anemia seen with ribavirin, senescence blunting of Interferon response on hepatocytes due to age-related oxidative stress

In addition to cost-effectiveness, many studies documented the safety and efficacy of Sofosbuvir as a component of combination therapy in the elderly population. Combination therapies included Sofosbuvir/ Daclatasvir, Sofosbuvir/Simeprevir, Sofosbuvir/Ribavirin [10, 41].

The sofosbuvir/ribavirin combination achieves high SVR rates in elderly patients, although a higher incidence of adverse events was observed. Most commonly reported adverse events to include pruritis and anemia. Nevertheless, the discontinuation rates were minimal [42].

Data on treatment with sofosbuvir plus simeprevir in elderly patients are limited. Ledipasvir/sofosbuvir treatment has very promising SVR12 rates in elderly patients age 65 years and older [10, 41].

As Sofosbuvir is renally cleared, renal function is a major determinant of Sofosbuvir in patients aged >64 years. Some studies demonstrated cirrhosis and baseline hemoglobin were the only independent predictors of severe adverse events in the elderly. Fatigue is the most common adverse event that was reported. The statement "Age per se should not be considered a contraindication, rather frailty, co-morbidities, and associated treatments should be carefully evaluated" remains valid for anti-HCV therapy [23, 32].

In summary, the current US FDA approved all-oral DAA regimens represent significant advances in elderly patients, as this group of patients has a faster progression of fibrosis and related complication compounded by polypharmacy in this traditionally difficult to treat group. Sofosbuvir can be safely used in elderly patients with HCV infection as a part of combination therapy to achieve SVR12, after considering frailty, renal function, co-morbidities, and drug to drug interaction [43, 44].

5. INDICATIONS AND USAGE

Sofosbuvir is only recommended with some combination of ribavirin, peginterferon-alfa, simeprevir, ledipasvir, daclatasvir, or velpatasvir [45, 46]. Cure rates are 30 to 97% depending on the type of hepatitis C virus involved. Sofosbuvir should not be used as a monotherapy as SVR may not be optimally achieved unless used in combination with other medications, although a single retrospective study demonstrated that seven days of sofosbuvir monotherapy only modestly reduces HCV RNA by 4.56 logs in individuals with HCV genotype1 [47]. Other drugs that can be used in combination with Sofosbuvir include other direct-acting antivirals (DAA), including the NS3/4A protease inhibitors (Simeprevir), the purine nucleoside analog (Ribavirin) and the NS5A inhibitors (Daclatasvir, Ledipasvir or Velpatasvir) [41, 48].

As per the recommendations formulated by the American Association for the Study of Liver Diseases and the Infectious Diseases Society of America for the management of hepatitis C, Sofosbuvir used in combination with other drugs is part of all first-line treatments for HCV genotypes 1, 2, 3, 4, 5, and 6, and is also part of some second-line treatments [41]. One reason for its efficacy against all HCV genotypes is it inhibits NS5B polymerase. This region NSB polymerase is well conserved across all the genotypes of HCV. It is efficacious if given as a component therapy in treatment naïve, treatment-experienced without cirrhosis or with compensated or decompensated cirrhosis. Also, efficacy has been demonstrated in patients with HIV/HCV coinfection and in patients who develop recurrent HCV infection post-transplantation [41].

There is published data available for its efficacy against HCV genotype 7 (Sofosbuvir in combination with Velpatasvir) that was isolated in Africa [49-52].

It is also used as a component of a combination antiviral regimen for patients with HCV/HIV -1 coinfection [10, 41].

5.1. Principles and Practice in Choosing a Sofosbuvir Based Regimen

Sofosbuvir-based regimens provide a higher cure rate, fewer side effects, and a two- to four-fold reduced duration of therapy [53-55]. Although the duration of therapy is ultimately decided by the stage of Cirrhosis, genotype, and other clinical circumstances. The usual duration of the combination therapy is around 12 weeks, although selected patients can be considered for as short as eight weeks to around 24 weeks. Peginterferon with or without sofosbuvir is no longer recommended in an initial HCV treatment [56].

Sofosbuvir, in combination with velpatasvir, is recommended for all genotypes with a cure rate greater than 90%, and close to 100% in most cases. The duration of treatment is typically 12 weeks [57].

For the treatment of genotypes 1, 4, 5, and six hepatitis C infections, Sofosbuvir can be used in combination with the viral NS5A inhibitor Ledipasvir [10, 41].

In genotype 2 and 3 HCV infections, Sofosbuvir can be used in combination with Daclatasvir. For the treatment of cases with cirrhosis or liver transplant patients, weight-based ribavirin is sometimes added [10, 41].

Compared to previous treatments, Sofosbuvir allows most people to be treated successfully without the use of Peginterferon, an injectable drug with severe side effects that is a key component of older drug combinations for the treatment of hepatitis C virus [58].

For people who have experienced treatment failure with some form of combination therapy for hepatitis C infection, one of the next possible steps would be retreatment with Sofosbuvir and either Ledipasvir or Daclatasvir, with or without weight-based ribavirin. At times, the combination of Sofosbuvir, Velpatasvir, and Voxilaprevir is also chosen. [34] The appropriate combination therapy should be chosen based on the genotype and the initially failed regimen, in addition to the general considerations like presence or absence of cirrhosis and if so compensated or decompensated. The duration can vary from 12-24 weeks. Unique patient population like (Pediatrics, geriatrics, Post-transplant, HIV co-infection) also need to be considered [10, 41].

6. CONTRAINDICATIONS

There are no specific contraindications for sofosbuvir when used alone. However, when used in combination with ribavirin or peginterferon alfa/ribavirin, or others, the contraindications applicable to these agents are applied [23].

7. SOFOSBUVIR ADVERSE EFFECTS

There are no hallmark toxicities associated with Sofosbuvir use. Side effects are observed when Sofosbuvir is administered as part of combination DAA, depending on the agent that is combined with it [23].

In combination with Ribavirin, most commonly reported side effects include fatigue and headache [32, 59].

In combination with Peginterferon alfa and ribavirin, most common adverse effects include fatigue, headache, nausea, insomnia, and anemia [32].

7.1. Asymptomatic Elevation of Enzymes

When given in combination with Peg IFN and ribavirin, some studies reported elevated bilirubin levels that peak at 1-2 weeks, returning to baseline by 4th-week post-treatment. Typically the transaminase levels are normal. These benign and transient elevations of bilirubin were even observed more so often in patients with HIV/HCV co-infection. Occasionally asymptomatic Creatinine kinase elevations of greater than or equal to ten times the upper limit of normal were observed in other studies.

Also Isolated, asymptomatic lipase elevation of greater than three times upper limit of normal was observed in some studies. When these enzyme elevations represent a subclinical injury, or a completely benign phenomenon remain to be answered. However, at this current time of publication, these benign elevations without accompanying clinical features is not an indication to discontinue therapy, rather heightened vigilance is suggested [32].

7.2. Reactivation of Hepatitis B

It must be emphasized that reactivation of Hepatitis B virus can occur when anti HCV therapy is started in a patient with Co-infection of Hepatitis B and C virus, esp if not receiving anti-HBV therapy. Some cases have resulted in fulminant hepatitis, hepatic failure, and death. Cases have been reported in patients who are HBsAg positive and also in patients with serologic evidence of resolved HBV infection (i.e., HBsAg negative and anti-HBc positive). HBV reactivation has also been reported in patients receiving certain immunosuppressant or chemotherapeutic agents; the risk of HBV reactivation associated with treatment with HCV direct-acting antivirals may be increased in these patients [60]. HBV reactivation is characterized as an abrupt increase in HBV replication manifesting as a rapid increase in serum HBV DNA level. In patients with resolved HBV infection, the reappearance of HBsAg can occur. Reactivation of HBV replication may be accompanied by hepatitis, i.e., increases in aminotransferase levels and, in severe cases, increases in bilirubin levels, liver failure, and death can occur. Hence, it is prudent to screen all patients with Hepatitis B virus infection before starting anti HCV therapy. Rather it is a boxed warning by the FDA [61].

Co-infected individuals usually have low or undetectable HBV DNA levels, which may be due to induction of types I and III interferons by HCV, both of which are active against HBV. This finding is in keeping with the observation that HBV reactivation related to interferon-based therapy for HCV typically occurred much later, usually after treatment.

With DAAs, rapid HCV suppression leads to reduced activation of the interferon cascade, allowing for enhanced HBV replication as early as four weeks into therapy [62].

The clinical outcome of increased HBV replication likely relates to the degree of immune control that predated therapy, which may explain why those with detectable HBV DNA seem to be at least at a somewhat higher risk [61, 62].

The FDA warning advises HBV DNA measurement even in those with resolved HBV infection who are HBsAg negative but anti-hepatitis B core (HBc) positive, although most if not all anti–HBc-positive individuals have replication-competent HBV DNA in the liver, the risk of reactivation is much lower in those who are HBsAg negative. This difference has been clearly shown in the setting of immunosuppression, with reactivation occurring in HBsAg-negative individuals only with profound immunosuppression (e.g., rituximab, stem cell transplantation) and extremely rare with lesser immunosuppression (e.g., solid tumor chemotherapy, steroids) [60].

Similarly, the risk of reactivation from anti-HCV therapy in HBsAg-negative patients is also very low. Since the initial FDA report, multiple studies, including a meta-analysis, have evaluated anti–HBc-positive/HBsAg-negative patients receiving DAAs with no reported cases of clinically significant reactivation in the absence of concomitant immunosuppression. This issue is important because a high proportion of HCV-infected individuals have been exposed to HBV, often through the same exposure that led to HCV infection [63].

All patients need to be screened for HBV before starting DAAs. For those who are HBsAg negative/anti–HBc positive, the risk is very low. It is not clear that HBV DNA is helpful and, as such, the American Association for the Study of Liver Diseases/Infectious Diseases Society of America and European Association for the Study of the Liver recommendation is to proceed with DAA therapy and reevaluate HBV only if ALT increases or fails to normalize on or after therapy [41].

For HBsAg-positive individuals meeting HBV treatment criteria at baseline, anti-HBV therapy should be initiated. Those with lower levels of

ALT and HBV DNA, Stratification by the presence of detectable HBV DNA may be a reasonable approach. Those with undetectable HBV DNA require ongoing monitoring, but may not require preemptive therapy. For those with detectable HBV DNA, although monitoring without treatment certainly is not unreasonable, given a >6% risk of clinically significant and potentially very severe reactivation, preemptive anti-HBV therapy may be warranted. Although the optimal duration of preemptive therapy is unknown, it seems reasonable to continue to SVR12. Importantly, whatever strategy is taken, continued monitoring after DAA completion and withdrawal of HBV therapy is required, because withdrawal flares are a concern [10, 41].

A proposed approach for HCV management in individuals with resolved or current HBV coinfection based on the risk of reactivation, the summary of which is as follows:

HBsAg-positive patients with positive baseline HBV DNA should be started on preemptive anti-HBV treatment until SVR12. HBsAg-positive patients with undetectable baseline HBV DNA should be either considered for preemptive anti-HBV treatment or monitored with ALT and HBV DNA until SVR12. HBsAg-negative/HBcAb-positive patients should be monitored with ALT alone until SVR12 and should be tested with HBsAg ± HBV DNA only if ALT increases or fails to normalize on therapy. Follow-up is required after stopping anti-HBV therapy owing to the risk of treatment withdrawal HBV flares [64, 65].

7.3. Toxicity

The highest documented dose of sofosbuvir was a single supratherapeutic dose of sofosbuvir 1200 mg administered to 59 healthy subjects. In that trial, there were no untoward effects observed at this dose level, and adverse events were similar in frequency and severity to those reported in the placebo and sofosbuvir 400 mg treatment groups [66].

At a dosage three times the maximum recommended dosage, Sofosbuvir does not prolong QTc to any clinically relevant extent. There is no specific antidote to overdosage. Treatment of overdose with sofosbuvir consists of general supportive measures, including monitoring of vital signs as well as observation of the clinical status of the patient. A 4-hour hemodialysis session would be expected to remove 18% of the administered dose [32].

Sofosbuvir was not genotoxic in a battery of in vitro or in vivo assays, including bacterial mutagenicity, chromosome aberration using human peripheral blood lymphocytes and in vivo mouse micronucleus assays [67].

Sofosbuvir had no effects on embryo-fetal viability or fertility when evaluated in rats. At the highest dose tested, AUC exposure to the predominant circulating metabolite GS-331007 was approximately eight times the exposure in humans at the recommended clinical dose [67].

8. Drug Interactions

Although widely successful, Hepatitis C therapy is still a challenge, especially in patients with multiple comorbidities. Therefore, special care and attention should be paid to drug interactions and individualized treatment strategies.

8.1. Amiodarone

In combination with Amiodarone, serious symptomatic bradycardia may be observed with symptoms consistent with low cardiac output state that include dizziness, lightheadedness, fatigue, tiredness, chest pain, and confusion that might require a pacemaker. The mechanism for this is unclear, but the interaction appears to be more pharmacodynamic rather than pharmacokinetic. Hence co-administration of Sofosbuvir and Amiodarone is not recommended. In patients without alternative, viable options, cardiac monitoring for at least the first two weeks should be strongly considered [68, 69]. Due to Amiodarone's long half-life, patients discontinuing Amiodarone just before starting Sofosbuvir should also undergo similar cardiac monitoring.

Alternatively, some case reports suggest the safety of Elbasvir/Grazoprevir use in patients taking Amiodarone. Although no cases of pharmacological interactions with Amiodarone for elbasvir/grazoprevir are known and the described interactions between sofosbuvir and amiodarone are most likely caused by a direct cardiotoxic effect of sofosbuvir rather than enzyme interactions, a potential risk due to a slight CYP3A4 inhibition by grazoprevir does exist. Grazoprevir in return can be affected by strong CYP3A4 inhibitors, and although amiodarone is known to only cause a slight CYP3A4 inhibition, drug interactions are often difficult to anticipate, especially in multimorbid patients [70, 71].

8.2. P-Glycoprotein (Permeability-Glycoproteins/MDR1) Related Drugs

Sofosbuvir is a substrate of P-glycoprotein, a transporter protein that pumps drugs and other substances from intestinal epithelium cells back into the gut. Therefore, inducers of intestinal P-glycoprotein (MDR1) efflux transporter, such as rifampicin, rifabutin, rifapentine, Carbamazepine, Oxcarbazepine, phenobarbitals, Phenytoin, Fosphenytoin and St. John's wort, Tipranavir could reduce the absorption of sofosbuvir and subsequently decreased conversion to an active metabolite [32, 72].

Drugs such as Daclatasvir, Eliglustat, Paritaprevir, Ritonavir, Sarecycline increase the level/effect of Sofosbuvir by its inhibitory action on P-glycoprotein [32, 72].

8.3. BCRP/ABCG2 Related Drugs

BCRP abbreviated for Breast cancer Resistance protein, also known as ABCG2 (ATP binding cassette sub-family G member 2) is an efflux transporter that serves two major drug transport functions. Firstly, it restricts the distribution of its substrates into organs such as the brain, testes, and placenta and across the GIT. Secondly, it eliminates its substrates from excretory org and, mediating both biliary and renal excretion, and occasionally, direct gut secretion. It is often co-expressed with MDR-1 [22].

Sofosbuvir is a substrate of efflux transporter BCRP and therefore drugs that inhibit this transporter like Acalabrutinib, Regorafenib, Safinamide, Stiripentol increases levels of Sofosbuvir. Drugs that induce BCRP like Apalutamide decrease the levels of Sofosbuvir. In summary, P-glycoprotein and BCRP inducers decrease the levels of sofosbuvir and P-glycoprotein, and BCRP inhibitors increase the levels of Sofosbuvir. [32, 72].

8.4. HIV Related Drugs

Sofosbuvir-based regimens should not be used with Tipranavir, as the latter can affect the P-glycoprotein [23]. It cannot be overemphasized that Sofosbuvir should not be co-administered with Elvitegravir/Cobicistat /emtricitabine/tenofovir disoproxil fumarate due to the drug to drug interactions via P-glycoproteins/BCRP [73].

There is no unique interaction between Sofosbuvir and HIV related drugs other than those associated with the efflux transporters. Nevertheless, it must be remembered that when choosing a regimen, drug to drug interactions related to all the components of the combination therapy must be considered. Following is a list of few examples describing the interactions between certain sofosbuvir-containing regimens and HIV related drugs.

Sofosbuvir/Velpatasvir should not be used with Efavirenz, Etravirine, or Nevirapine. Velptasvir in this regimen can cause elevation of Tenofovir disoproxil fumarate levels. C. This concomitant use mandates consideration of renal function and should be avoided in those with an eGFR <60 mL/min [73].

Ledipasvir/Sofosbuvir can be used with most antiretrovirals. Because this therapy increases Tenofovir levels when given as Tenofovir disoproxil fumarate, concomitant use mandates consideration of renal function and should be avoided in those with an eGFR <60 mL/min [23, 73].

Sofosbuvir/Velpatasvir/Voxilaprevir should not be used with Ritonavir-boosted atazanavir, efavirenz, etravirine, or nevirapine. This therapy can be considered with drugs that do not have substantial interactions like Dolutergravir, Emtricitabine, Enfuvirtide, Lamivudine, Rilpivirine, and Raltegravir [32, 73].

The interaction between Sofosbuvir and some other drugs, such as darunavir/ritonavir, efavirenz, emtricitabine, raltegravir, rilpivirine, tenofovir disoproxil, Atazanavir, Dolutegravir, Elvitegravir/cobicistat, Lopinavir/Ritonavir were evaluated in clinical trials, and no dose adjustment is needed for any of these drugs. However, all the components of the combination therapy must be checked for interactions [73].

8.5. CYP 3A4 Inducers

Sofosbuvir by itself is not a CYP substrate, inhibitor or inducer and therefore low potential for interactions with drugs that affect CYP enzyme system. One is advised to check the interactions with all of the components of combination therapy when choosing a regimen.

For example, Co-administration of Sofosbuvir/Velpatasavir with drugs that induce CYP 3A4 is not recommended as this may lead to loss of Anti HCV efficacy. Some examples of Anti-HIV drugs that induce CYP 3A4 include Etravirine and Nevirapine [32].

8.6. Warfarin Interaction

Fluctuations in INR values may occur in patients receiving Warfarin concomitant with HCV treatment. Frequent monitoring of INR values is recommended during treatment, and post-treatment follow up. Some studies indicate warfarin toxicity and other studies reported a clinically significant reduction in warfarin dose-response and possibly sub-therapeutic levels of anticoagulation. Hence, a perfect conclusion cannot be drawn as of now, and frequent monitoring of INR is essential [74].

8.7. Calcineurin Inhibitors (Post Transplant Patients)

Cyclosporin increases the Sofosbuvir exposure (4.5 increase in AUC), but GS-331007 metabolite is unchanged, and because of the high therapeutic index, no prior dose adjustment is required [32].

No drug to drug interaction was observed between Sofosbuvir and Tacrolimus [75].

8.8. Acid-Reducing Medications

Anti-Secretory therapy can decrease the effectiveness of some patients and could prevent a successful cure.

Though Sofosbuvir per-se is not affected by the acid in the stomach, the other components (another antiviral) of the combination therapy are affected. Hence following is a guideline for dosing adjustment. Also, it is prudent not to exceed a "recommended dose" of acid-reducing drugs [76].

8.8.1. For Sofosbuvir/Velpatasvir

Antacids (Aluminium, Magnesium or Calcium-containing antacids) to be taken 4 hours apart.

H2 blockers: May be taken together with the DAA therapy or 12 hours apart.

Proton Pump Inhibitors (PPI): It is best to avoid PPI if Sofosbuvir/Velapatsvir is being considered. In case of no alternatives, PPI should be taken 4 hours after Sofosbuvir/Velpatasvir. Sofosbuvir/Velpatasvir to be taken with food [76].

8.8.2. For Sofosbuvir /Ledipasvir

Antacids (Aluminium, Magnesium or Calcium-containing antacids) to be taken 4 hours apart.

H2 blockers: May be taken together with the DAA therapy or 12 hours apart.

PPI: It is best to avoid PPI if Sofosbuvir/Ledipasvir is being considered. In case of no alternatives, PPI should be taken at the same time as Sofosbuvir/Ledipasvir, in the morning after overnight fasting (On an empty stomach) [76].

Recommended doses of anti-secretary therapy: While on anti-viral therapy, it is recommended not to exceed a certain "recommended dose" of these drugs. Following is a general guideline of this recommended dose.

H2 blockers: Cimetidine (400mg PO Q12), Famotidine (40mg Q12), Nizatidine (300mg Q12), Ranitidine (300 mg Q12 hrs).

PPI: Esomeprazole (20 mg once daily), Lansoprazole (15 mg Once daily), Omeprazole (20 mg Once daily), Pantoprazole (40 mg once daily), Rabeprazole (20 mg Once daily) [76].

Methadone: No dose adjustment is required for Sofosbuvir [32].

8.8.3. Other Intracellularly Acting Drugs

The intracellular metabolic activation pathway of sofosbuvir is mediated by generally low affinity and high capacity hydrolase and nucleotide phosphorylation pathways that are unlikely to be affected by concomitant drugs that act intracellularly [32].

9. RESISTANCE TO SOFOSBUVIR

Sofosbuvir has a high genetic barrier to resistance in contrast to NS5A and NS3/4A inhibitors. This is in part to the highly conserved catalytic site region where nucleotides bind, making substitutions in this region extremely rare. Additionally, any such substitution would likely render the virus replication-incompetent [23].

Though it is believed that Sofosbuvir has a high genetic barrier to resistance, many RAVs or resistant associated substitutions have been described in the literature and reported in patients who relapsed to Sofosbuvir-based treatment [77, 78]. Some of the Resistance-associated substitutions include S282T, L159F, V321A, and C316N/H/F, M289L as reported in cell culture and pooled analysis assays from next-generation nucleotide sequencing of NS5B genotypic data with the assay cutoff of 1%. Though it has been believed that these associated resistance substitutions may revert to original prototype if the selection pressure is removed, it must not be taken for granted, and persistence and rather transmission of these RASs are also described. [106]. It is also interesting to note that sometimes these RASs may leave a genetic footprint at the level of RNA that may be detected at a later date yielding a timeline for the development of this mutation [28].

Although no resistance testing is recommended at this time before initiating Sofosbuvir, as it is usually given as a combination therapy, resistance testing should be considered depending on the combination therapy and the genotype of HCV. For example, NS5A RAS testing should be considered for genotype 1a infected; treatment-experienced patients with or without cirrhosis being considered for Ledipasvir/Sofosbuvir. NS5A RAS testing is recommended for genotype three infected, treatment-naive patients with cirrhosis or treatment-experienced patients without cirrhosis being considered for Sofosbuvir/Velpatasvir or Sofosbuvir/ Daclatasvir. Some guidelines suggest the addition of weight-based ribavirin if the RAS is found to be Y93H [10, 41].

9.1. Cross-Resistance

HCV replicons expressing the sofosbuvir-associated resistance substitution S282T were susceptible to NS5A inhibitors and ribavirin. HCV replicons expressing the associated ribavirin substitutions T390I and F415Y were susceptible to sofosbuvir. Sofosbuvir was active against HCV replicons with NS3/4A protease inhibitor, NS5B non-nucleoside inhibitor, and NS5A inhibitor-resistant variants [77].

CONCLUSION

Sofosbuvir is a prodrug based on Uridine analog. After crossing the plasma membrane, this prodrug undergoes cleavage and subsequent phosphorylation yields the active "Triphosphate" form. This active form designated GS-461203 competes with uridine triphosphate for incorporation into HCV RNA by NS5B polymerase, thus inhibiting HCV replication. Later Sofosbuvir is metabolized by hydrolysis to an inactive form and eliminated in the urine via tubular secretion and glomerular filtration. As NS5B polymerase region is well conserved across genotypes, Sofosbuvir is active against all HCV genotypes.

The dose of Sofosbuvir is 400mg once daily and primarily used in combination with other anti HCV drugs (NS3/4A protease inhibitors, NS5A inhibitors, purine nucleoside analogs). Sofosbuvir exhibits near-linear kinetics across a range of doses. The available data suggests no dose modification in conditions with increased bioavailability as seen in either decompensated cirrhosis or after a high-fat meal. This is probably because of the drugs high therapeutic index. In contrast, the pharmacokinetics of sofosbuvir is significantly affected by the severity of renal impairment. Several studies suggested that Sofosbuvir be not used in patients with eGFR of less than 30 ml/min/1.73m2 and those with ESRD requiring dialysis until further data about the dose modification is available. Dose modification may not be required for eGFR > 30 ml/min/1.73m2. Sofosbuvir is currently not approved in children, although safety and efficacy have been demonstrated in certain studies for children more than 6 Years of age. The pharmacokinetic profile appears to be similar in the geriatric population.

There are no hallmark toxicities associated with Sofosbuvir use. Side effects may be observed due to the co-administered drug in the combination of anti HCV therapy. As Sofosbuvir is not a CYP substrate, inducer, or inhibitor, it has a low potential for drug interaction. However, Sofosbuvir is a substrate for efflux transporters Pgp and BCRP, and thus caution should be exercised in patients taking potent inducers of these transporters (Rifampicin, Phenytoin, Carbamazepine, St John's wart). For an unclear mechanism, Sofosbuvir containing DAA treatments have been associated with fatal cardiac arrest, bradycardia requiring pacemaker insertion in patients taking Amiodarone. This could be due to pharmacodynamic interaction.

Lastly, despite poor fidelity and lack of proofreading activity of HCV NS5B polymerase enzyme (thus allowing for spontaneous viral mutations, so-called Resistant associated variants- RAVs), Nucleotide NS5B polymerase inhibitors like Sofobuvir have a high genetic barrier to resistance, unlike the other classes of anti HCV medications. Three or more RAV is required for a full resistance. However, certain RAV (S282T, L159F, V321A, and C316N/H/F) have been reported in patients who relapsed on sofosbuvir-based treatment.

REFERENCES

[1] CDC Viral Hepatitis. https://www.cdc.gov/hepatitis/hcv/hcvfaq.htm#section1.
[2] "FDA approves first combination pill to treat hepatitis C". Archived from the original on 2015-05-04.
[3] Herper, M. F., 2014). "Gilead's Hepatitis C Pill Takes Off Like a Rocket." *Forbes.* Archived from the original on August 31, 2017.
[4] "Essential Medicines WHO Model List, 19th edition" (PDF). *World Health Organization.* April 2015. Archived (PDF) from the original on 2015-05-13.
[5] Messina, J. P., et al., Global distribution and prevalence of hepatitis C virus genotypes. *Hepatology,* 2015. **61**(1): p. 77-87.
[6] Tang, H. and H. Grisé, Cellular and molecular biology of HCV infection and hepatitis. *Clinical Science,* 2009. **117**(2): p. 49-65.

[7] Alter, H. J., HCV natural history: the retrospective and prospective in perspective. *Journal of hepatology*, 2005. **43**(4): p. 550-552.
[8] Neumann-Haefelin, C., et al., Dominant influence of an HLA-B27 restricted CD8$^+$ T cell response in mediating HCV clearance and evolution. *Hepatology*, 2006. **43**(3): p. 563-572.
[9] Parfieniuk, A., J. Jaroszewicz, and R. Flisiak, Specifically targeted antiviral therapy for hepatitis C virus. *World journal of gastroenterology: WJG*, 2007. **13**(43): p. 5673.
[10] European Association for the Study of the Liver (EASL). *Recommendations on treatment of hepatitis C* 2016. Available: www.easleu/research/our-contributions/clinical-practice-guidelines/ detail/easl-recommendations-on-treatment-of-hepatitis-c-2016.
[11] Asselah, T. and P. Marcellin, Direct acting antivirals for the treatment of chronic hepatitis C: one pill a day for tomorrow. *Liver International*, 2012. **32**: p. 88-102.
[12] Ghany, M. G., et al., An update on treatment of genotype 1 chronic hepatitis C virus infection: 2011 practice guideline by the American Association for the Study of Liver Diseases. *Hepatology*, 2011. **54**(4): p. 1433-1444.
[13] Koff, R., the efficacy and safety of sofosbuvir, a novel, oral nucleotide NS 5B polymerase inhibitor, in the treatment of chronic hepatitis C virus infection. *Alimentary pharmacology & therapeutics*, 2014. **39**(5): p. 478-487.
[14] Keating, G. M. and A. Vaidya, Sofosbuvir: first global approval. *Drugs*, 2014. **74**(2): p. 273-282.
[15] Lok, A. S.-F., HCV NS5A inhibitors in development. *Clinics in liver disease*, 2013. **17**(1): p. 111-121.
[16] Herbst, D. A. and K. R. Reddy, NS5A inhibitor, daclatasvir, for the treatment of chronic hepatitis C virus infection. *Expert opinion on investigational drugs*, 2013. **22**(10): p. 1337-1346.
[17] Sagnelli, E., et al., Resistance detection and re-treatment options in hepatitis C virus-related chronic liver diseases after DAA-treatment failure. *Infection*, 2018: p. 1-23.

[18] Murakami, E., et al., Mechanism of activation of PSI-7851 and its diastereoisomer PSI-7977. *Journal of biological chemistry*, 2010. **285**(45): p. 34337-34347.
[19] Fung, A., et al., Efficiency of incorporation and chain termination determines the inhibition potency of 2′-modified nucleotide analogs against hepatitis C virus polymerase. *Antimicrobial agents and chemotherapy*, 2014. **58**(7): p. 3636-3645.
[20] Ma, H., et al., Characterization of the metabolic activation of hepatitis C virus nucleoside inhibitor β-d-2′-deoxy-2′-fluoro-2′-C-methylcytidine (PSI-6130) and identification of a novel active 5′-triphosphate species. *Journal of Biological Chemistry*, 2007. **282**(41): p. 29812-29820.
[21] Dinnendahl V, F. U., eds. (2015). *Arzneistoff-Profile [Drug's profile]* (in German). 9 (28 ed.). Eschborn, Germany: Govi Pharmazeutischer Verlag. ISBN 978-3-7741-9846-3.
[22] Kirby, B. J., et al., Pharmacokinetic, pharmacodynamic, and drug-interaction profile of the hepatitis C virus NS5B polymerase inhibitor sofosbuvir. *Clinical Pharmacokinetics*, 2015. **54**(7): p. 677-690.
[23] *Goodman & Gilman's the pharmacological basis of therapeutics.* Brunton, L. L. K., Björn C; Hilal-Dandan, Randa. Thirteenth edition. New York: McGraw Hill Medical, [2018].
[24] Goldberg, D., et al., Changes in the prevalence of hepatitis C virus infection, nonalcoholic steatohepatitis, and alcoholic liver disease among patients with cirrhosis or liver failure on the waitlist for liver transplantation. *Gastroenterology*, 2017. **152**(5): p. 1090-1099. e1.
[25] Curry, M. P., et al., Sofosbuvir and velpatasvir for HCV in patients with decompensated cirrhosis. *New England Journal of Medicine*, 2015. **373**(27): p. 2618-2628.
[26] Manns, M., et al., Ledipasvir and sofosbuvir plus ribavirin in patients with genotype 1 or 4 hepatitis C virus infection and advanced liver disease: a multicentre, open-label, randomised, phase 2 trial. *The Lancet Infectious Diseases*, 2016. **16**(6): p. 685-697.

[27] Poordad, F., et al., Daclatasvir with sofosbuvir and ribavirin for hepatitis C virus infection with advanced cirrhosis or post-liver transplantation recurrence. *Hepatology,* 2016. **63**(5): p. 1493-1505.
[28] Foster, G. R., et al., Impact of direct acting antiviral therapy in patients with chronic hepatitis C and decompensated cirrhosis. *J Hepatol*, 2016. **64**(6): p. 1224-31.
[29] Desnoyer, A., et al., Pharmacokinetics, safety and efficacy of a full dose sofosbuvir-based regimen given daily in hemodialysis patients with chronic hepatitis C. *J Hepatol,* 2016. **65**(1): p. 40-47.
[30] Saxena, V., et al., Safety and efficacy of sofosbuvir-containing regimens in hepatitis C-infected patients with impaired renal function. *Liver Int,* 2016. **36**(6): p. 807-16.
[31] Nazario, H. E., M. Ndungu, and A. A. Modi, Sofosbuvir and simeprevir in hepatitis C genotype 1-patients with end-stage renal disease on haemodialysis or GFR <30 ml/min. *Liver International,* 2016. **36**(6): p. 798-801.
[32] *SOVALDI* [Package Insert]. Foster City, CA: Gilead Sciences Inc; 2013. Available from Drugs@FDA: http://www.accessdata.fda.gov/drugsat-fda_docs/label/2017/204671s007lbl.pdf.
[33] Copegus (Ribavirin, USP Tablets) *"Medication Guide"* (PDF). Roche. https://www.accessdata.fda.gov/drugsatfda_docs/label/"2005/021511s012lbl.pdf.
[34] *FDA.* https://www.fda.gov/news-events/press-announcements/fda-approves-two-hepatitis-c-drugs-pediatric-patients
[35] Ghobrial, C., et al., Is sofosbuvir/ledipasvir safe for the hearts of children with hepatitis C virus? *Dig Liver Dis*, 2019. **51**(2): p. 258-262.
[36] Murray, K. F., et al., Safety and Efficacy of Ledipasvir–Sofosbuvir with or Without Ribavirin for Chronic Hepatitis C in Children Ages 6-11. *Hepatology,* 2018. **68**(6): p. 2158-2166.
[37] Pariente, A., et al., Effects of Age on Treatment of Chronic Hepatitis C with Direct Acting Antivirals. *Ann Hepatol*, 2018. **18**(1): p. 193-202.

[38] Sherigar, J. M., et al., Clinical efficacy and tolerability of direct-acting antivirals in elderly patients with chronic hepatitis C. *Eur J Gastroenterol Hepatol*, 2017. **29**(7): p. 767-776.
[39] Younossi, Z., et al., the Use of All Oral Regimens for Treatment of Chronic Hepatitis C (chc) Coupled with Birth Cohort Screening Is Highly Cost Effective: The Health and Economic Impact on the Us Population: 116. *Hepatology*, 2014. **60**: p. 256A.
[40] Rein, D., et al., P785 Projected Health And Economic Impact of Hepatitis C on the United States Veterans Administration Health System From 2014 TO 2024. *Journal of Hepatology*, 2014. **60**(1): p. S332.
[41] *AASLD HCV guidelines*. https://www.hcvguidelines.org/.
[42] Zeuzem, S., et al., Sofosbuvir and ribavirin in HCV genotypes 2 and 3. *New England Journal of Medicine*, 2014. **370**(21): p. 1993-2001.
[43] Rheem, J., V. Sundaram, and S. Saab, Antiviral therapy in elderly patients with hepatitis C virus infection. *Gastroenterology & hepatology*, 2015. **11**(5): p. 294.
[44] Su, F., et al., Direct-acting antivirals are effective for chronic hepatitis C treatment in elderly patients: a real-world study of 17 487 patients. *European journal of gastroenterology & hepatology*, 2017. **29**(6): p. 686-693.
[45] "*Sofosbuvir (Sovaldi)-Treatment-Hepatitis C Online.*" https://www.hepatitisc.uw.edu/page/treatment/drugs/sofosbuvir-drug.
[46] FDA, News Release (June 28, 2016). "*FDA approves Epclusa for treatment of chronic Hepatitis C virus infection.*" Archived from the original on June 3, 2017.
[47] Lawitz, E., et al., Sofosbuvir in combination with peginterferon alfa-2a and ribavirin for non-cirrhotic, treatment-naive patients with genotypes 1, 2, and 3 hepatitis C infection: a randomised, double-blind, phase 2 trial. *The Lancet infectious diseases*, 2013. **13**(5): p. 401-408.
[48] Rodriguez-Torres, M., et al., Sofosbuvir (GS-7977) plus peginterferon/ribavirin in treatment-naive patients with HCV

genotype 1: a randomized, 28-day, dose-ranging trial. *Journal of hepatology*, 2013. **58**(4): p. 663-668.

[49] Schreiber, J., et al., Treatment of a patient with genotype 7 hepatitis C virus infection with sofosbuvir and velpatasvir. H*epatology*, 2016. **64**(3): p. 983-985.

[50] Smith, D. B., et al., Expanded classification of hepatitis C virus into 7 genotypes and 67 subtypes: updated criteria and genotype assignment web resource. *Hepatology,* 2014. **59**(1): p. 318-327.

[51] Hedskog, C., et al., Genotype-and subtype-independent full-genome sequencing assay for hepatitis C virus. *Journal of clinical microbiology,* 2015. **53**(7): p. 2049-2059.

[52] Murphy, D. G., et al., Hepatitis C virus genotype 7, a new genotype originating from central Africa. *Journal of clinical microbiology*, 2015. **53**(3): p. 967-972.

[53] Tran, T. T., A review of standard and newer treatment strategies in hepatitis C. *Am J Manag Care,* 2012. **18**(14 Suppl): p. S340-349.

[54] Berden, F., et al., Dutch guidance for the treatment of chronic hepatitis C virus infection in a new therapeutic era. *Neth J Med,* 2014. **72**(8): p. 388-400.

[55] Cholongitas, E. and G. V. Papatheodoridis, Sofosbuvir: a novel oral agent for chronic hepatitis C. *Annals of Gastroenterology: Quarterly Publication of the Hellenic Society of Gastroenterology*, 2014. **27**(4): p. 331.

[56] Yau, A. H. and E. M. Yoshida, Hepatitis C drugs: the end of the pegylated interferon era and the emergence of all-oral interferon-free antiviral regimens: a concise review. *Can J Gastroenterol Hepatol*, 2014. **28**(8): p. 445-51.

[57] "EPCLUSA (sofosbuvir and velpatasvir) Prescribing information" (PDF). *Gilead Sciences, Inc.* Archived (PDF) from the original on March 2019.

[58] Calvaruso, V., M. Mazza, and P. L. Almasio, Pegylated-interferon-alpha(2a) in clinical practice: how to manage patients suffering from side effects. *Expert Opin Drug Saf*, 2011. **10**(3): p. 429-35.

[59] Zeuzem, S., et al., Sofosbuvir and Ribavirin in HCV Genotypes 2 and 3. *New England Journal of Medicine*, 2014. **370**(21): p. 1993-2001.
[60] Paul, S., et al., Hepatitis B Virus Reactivation and Prophylaxis during Solid Tumor Chemotherapy: A Systematic Review and Meta-analysis. *Ann Intern Med*, 2016. **164**(1): p. 30-40.
[61] Chen, G., et al., Hepatitis B reactivation in hepatitis B and C coinfected patients treated with antiviral agents: A systematic review and meta-analysis. *Hepatology*, 2017. **66**(1): p. 13-26.
[62] Meissner, E. G., et al., Endogenous intrahepatic IFNs and association with IFN-free HCV treatment outcome. *J Clin Invest*, 2014. **124**(8): p. 3352-63.
[63] Sulkowski, M. S., et al., No Evidence of Reactivation of Hepatitis B Virus Among Patients Treated With Ledipasvir-Sofosbuvir for Hepatitis C Virus Infection. *Clin Infect Dis*, 2016. **63**(9): p. 1202-1204.
[64] Liu, C. J., et al., Efficacy of Ledipasvir and Sofosbuvir Treatment of HCV Infection in Patients Coinfected With HBV. *Gastroenterology*, 2018. **154**(4): p. 989-997.
[65] Bersoff-Matcha, S. J., et al., Hepatitis B Virus Reactivation Associated With Direct-Acting Antiviral Therapy for Chronic Hepatitis C Virus: A Review of Cases Reported to the U.S. Food and Drug Administration Adverse Event Reporting System. *Ann Intern Med*, 2017. **166**(11): p. 792-798.
[66] *Daily Med*, Current Medical Information for Sovaldi (Sofosbuvir) Tablet. http://dailymed.nlm.nih.gov/dailymed/drugInfo.cfm?setid=80beab2c-396e-4a37-a4dc-40fdb62859cf.
[67] "Sofosbuvir label" (PDF). *FDA*. August 2015. Archived (PDF) from the original on March 2019.
[68] FDA Drug Safety Podcast FDA warns of serious slowing of the heart rate when antiarrhythmic drug amiodarone is used with hepatitis C treatments containing sofosbuvir (Harvoni) or Sovaldi in combination with another direct-acting antiviral drug. https://www.fda.gov/downloads/Drugs/DrugSafety/UCM439492.pdf

[69] *European Medicines Agency EMA recommends avoidance of certain hepatitis C medicines and amiodarone together.* http://www.ema. europa.eu/ docs/ en_GB/ document_library/ Press_release/ 2015/ 04/ WC500186152.pdf.

[70] Back, D.J. and D.M. Burger, Interaction between amiodarone and sofosbuvir-based treatment for hepatitis C virus infection: potential mechanisms and lessons to be learned. *Gastroenterology*, 2015. **149**(6): p. 1315-7.

[71] Weiss, L., et al., Elbasvir/Grazoprevir, an Alternative in Antiviral Hepatitis C Therapy in Patients under Amiodarone Treatment. *Case Rep Gastroenterol*, 2018. **12**(1): p. 92-98.

[72] 2019., *S.l.P.F.A.A.P.f.t.o.o.M.*

[73] Karageorgopoulos, D. E., et al., Drug interactions between antiretrovirals and new or emerging direct-acting antivirals in HIV/hepatitis C virus coinfection. *Curr Opin Infect Dis*, 2014. **27**(1): p. 36-45.

[74] DeCarolis, D. D., et al., Evaluation of a Potential Interaction between New Regimens to Treat Hepatitis C and Warfarin. *Ann Pharmacother*, 2016. **50**(11): p. 909-917.

[75] Kiser, J. J., J. R. Burton, Jr., and G. T. Everson, Drug-drug interactions during antiviral therapy for chronic hepatitis C. *Nat Rev Gastroenterol Hepatol*, 2013. **10**(10): p. 596-606.

[76] DeVreese, L. et al., Influence of Proton Pump Inhibitors and H2 Receptor Antagonists on Direct Acting Antiviral HCV Sustained Virologic Response. *Journal of Hepatology*, 2016. **64**(2): p. S790.

[77] Donaldson, E. F., et al., Clinical evidence and bioinformatics characterization of potential hepatitis C virus resistance pathways for sofosbuvir. Hepatology, 2015. **61**(1): p. 56-65.

[78] Hedskog, C. et al., Evolution of the HCV viral population from a patient with S282T detected at relapse after sofosbuvir monotherapy. *J Viral Hepat*, 2015. **22**(11): p. 871-81.

In: The Pharmacological Guide to Sofosbuvir ISBN: 978-1-53616-476-3
Editor: Vijay Gayam © 2019 Nova Science Publishers, Inc.

Chapter 2

SOFOSBUVIR IN NON-CIRRHOTIC PATIENTS WITH CHRONIC HEPATITIS C INFECTION

Amrendra Kumar Mandal[1,*], Benjamin Tiongson[1], Eric O. Then[2], Vijay Gayam[1] and Vinaya Gaduputi[2]

[1]Department of Internal Medicine, Interfaith Medical Center,
Brooklyn, NY, US
[2] Department of Internal Medicine, St. Barnabas Hospital Health System
Bronx, NY, US

ABSTRACT

Hepatitis C affects more than 71 million around the world and is one of the major causes of chronic liver disease worldwide. Management options for patients infected with chronic hepatitis C have evolved over the last few years. Introduction of newer direct-acting antivirals has revolutionized the treatment of this disease. Amongst all direct-acting antivirals, nucleoside inhibitors have been the most promising agent. Sofosbuvir (GS-7977), is a recently approved nucleotide analog and is a highly potent inhibitor of the NS5B polymerase in the Hepatitis C virus. Studies have shown this drug to have high efficacy either as dual therapy

[*] Corresponding Author's E-mail: Amandal@interfaithmedical.com

in conjunction with or without ribavirin or as triple therapy with either NS5A inhibitors or a protease inhibitor. Efficacy of sofosbuvir has also been established in various clinical trials like PROTON, ELECTRON, FUSION, POSITRON. Furthermore, it has a good safety profile with few mild to moderate adverse effects, and it is generally well-tolerated. Due to these reasons, sofosbuvir has been utilized as the backbone in a variety of combination regimens for the treatment of chronic hepatitis C and is the most widely used drug currently in the market to date.

Keywords: sofosbuvir, hepatitis C virus, NS5B polymerase, direct-acting antivirals, adverse effects

ABBREVIATIONS

HCV	Hepatitis C virus
WHO	World Health Organization
HCC	Hepatocellular Carcinoma
SVR	Sustained Virologic Response
CHC	Chronic Hepatitis C
FDA	Food and Drug Association
DAA	Direct-Acting Antivirals
Peg-IFN	pegylated interferon
RNA	Ribonucleic acid
AASLD	American Association for the Study of Liver Disease
IDSA	Infectious Disease Society of America
HIV	Human Immunodeficiency Virus

1. INTRODUCTION

The World Health Organization's (WHO) goals of significantly reducing morbidity and mortality rates from the Hepatitis C Virus (HCV) by 2030 requires a comprehensive effort to identify and treat all those that are infected [1]. Approximately 500,000 people die each year, primarily in lower to middle-income countries, from HCV-related complications [2].

Chronic HCV infection is also a common cause of hepatocellular carcinoma (HCC) and cirrhosis [3]. As a result, the eradication of HCV is an important endpoint as the sustained virological response (SVR) has been associated with the reversal of hepatic fibrosis and decreased rates of HCC [4, 5]. Table 1 shows the modifiable and non-modifiable risk factors for the progression of fibrosis.

The development of an effective antiviral therapy was considered a challenge before the advent of direct-acting antivirals (DAA), owing to some typical features making Chronic Hepatitis C (CHC) difficult to treat (e.g., genotypic variation, associated resistance variants, pre-existing liver conditions). However, the approval of the NS34A protease inhibitors boceprevir and telaprevir by the US Food and Drug Association (FDA), heralded the beginning of first-generation of DAA and marked a breakthrough in CHC treatment [6]. The addition of the protease inhibitors to pegylated-interferon (peg-IFN) and ribavirin combination increased the SVR rates between 66% and 75% in treatment-naive patients with chronic HCV genotype-1 infection. This combination was also associated with increased adverse events. Moreover, therapies based on both telaprevir and boceprevir had the disadvantages of high pill burdens, complicated dosing strategies, and a very low genetic barrier to resistance, which restricted their use [7].

In 2013, the US FDA approved sofosbuvir (previously known as GS-7977) for the treatment of CHC. Sofosbuvir is a (prototype) nucleotide analog antiviral, which acts as an inhibitor of HCV-specific NS5B ribonucleic acid polymerase (RNA). It has a good safety profile, has activity against all genotypes, and is being used as the first interferon-free treatment regimen option for CHC [8, 9]. Notably, with several new treatments on the horizon, there is hope that eventually the goal of complete eradication of HCV can be achieved.

2. NATURAL HISTORY OF THE HEPATITIS C VIRUS

Acute infection with HCV is usually asymptomatic, and is therefore frequently under-diagnosed and underestimated [10]. Acute HCV infection is usually transmitted through blood, although rarely, it is possible to transfer the disease via a sexual route [11]. The incubation period from infection to onset of symptoms can range from 2 to 12 weeks, with an average of 6–7 weeks [12]. Serum HCV RNA is detectable within 7–21 days after an acute infection, can be detected at the onset of jaundice in titers of 105–107 copies/mL. Aminotransferase levels are elevated between 14 and 28 days after infection, and anti-HCV becomes detectable approximately 60 days (varies from 20 to 150 days) after the onset of infection [13].

HCV is deemed chronic once HCV RNA has persisted for more than six months. A spontaneous clearance occurs within the first six months in only about 20% to 50% of patients. This outcome also depends partially on the clinical findings; it was noted in one study that patients with jaundice are more likely to clear acute HCV infection [14]. Based on initial studies from tertiary referral centers, it was estimated that liver cirrhosis would develop in about 15% to 30% of HCV-infected patients within 10 to 20 years, and some of these cases will progress to HCC. Consequently, HCV-induced chronic liver disease is recognized as the leading indication for orthotopic liver transplantation [15].

3. THE GOAL OF TREATMENT FOR HCV

The primary goal of antiviral therapy in patients with chronic hepatitis C is to reduce all-cause mortality and hepatic adverse consequences, like end-stage liver disease and HCC [16]. Viral eradication is determined by SVR, which is defined as undetectable HCV RNA following completion of therapy in serum and plasma [17]. SVR is generally associated with normalization of liver enzymes and improvement or disappearance of liver necroinflammation and fibrosis in patients without cirrhosis.

Table 1. Factors associated with accelerated fibrosis progression

Host	Viral
Non-modifiable Fibrosis stage Inflammation grade Older age at the time of infection Male sex Organ transplant ***Modifiable*** Alcohol consumption Nonalcoholic fatty liver disease Obesity Insulin resistance	Genotype 3 infection Co-infection with hepatitis B virus or HIV

Source: Hepatitis C Guidance 2018 Update: AASLD-IDSA Recommendations for Testing, Managing, and Treating Hepatitis C Virus Infection.

4. WHEN AND WHOM TO INITIATE HCV THERAPY

According to the American Association for the Study of Liver Diseases- Infectious Disease Society of America (AASLD-IDSA), treatment is recommended for all patients with chronic HCV infection, except those with a short life expectancy that cannot be remediated by treatment, liver transplantation or directed therapy [16]. Regardless of the strong recommendation for treatment of almost all HCV infected patients, patient education, and pretreatment assessment of their understanding of treatment goals is crucial for adherence and successful management. Establishment of good rapport between physician and patient remains important for optimal outcomes with DAA therapies [16]. Recommended pretreatment assessments include evaluation for advanced fibrosis using either liver biopsy, imaging, or non-invasive markers to facilitate decision making.

5. CLINICAL BENEFIT OF CURE

Treatment of HCV and achieving SVR has numerous direct and indirect health benefits. Patients experience a decrease in liver inflammation as reflected in better aminotransferase levels, and a reduction in the rate of liver fibrosis progression [18]. Furthermore, there is also marked improvement of advanced liver disease signs and symptoms, including patients having portal hypertension and splenomegaly. Risk of liver cancer (HCC) is reduced by > 70% upon achievement of SVR, and patients with non-Hodgkin's lymphoma and other lymphoproliferative disorders achieve partial or complete transmission after the documented success of HCV treatment [19-21].

Due to the numerous benefits associated with successful HCV treatment, it is imperative that health care providers focus on achieving SVR on all patients, preferably in the early stages of treatment, to reduce all-cause mortality and overall improvement of the quality of life of the patient [22, 23].

6. INITIAL TREATMENT OF HCV INFECTION

Initial treatment of HCV infection includes patients with CHC who have not been previously treated with IFN, peg-IFN, ribavirin, or any HCV DAA agent. Recommended treatment regimens for CHC in non-cirrhotics are summarized in Table 2.

7. SOFOSBUVIR-BASED TREATMENT REGIMENS BY GENOTYPE

Sofosbuvir should be administered at the dose of 400 mg (one tablet) once per day, with or without food. It is most useful when in combination with other DAAs and it is active on all the HCV genotypes, although there were studies had identified an S282T mutation reducing the susceptibility of sofosbuvir [24]. Regardless, clinical studies have consistently yielded a high SVR rate, and in one study, it was found that the S282T mutation was rare, implying a high resistance barrier [25]. Renal clearance is the major elimination pathway, and the majority of the sofosbuvir dose recovered in urine is the dephosphorylation-derived nucleoside metabolite GS-331007 (78%), while 3.5% is recovered as Sofosbuvir [24].

7.1. HCV Genotype 1

Four highly potent DAA combination regimens are recommended for patients with genotype 1 infection with comparable efficacy while another four regimens are classified as alternatives because of limited supporting data.

7.1.1. Ledipasvir/Sofosbuvir
The fixed-dose combination of ledipasvir (90 mg)/sofosbuvir (400 mg) was approved by the FDA for the treatment of HCV genotype 1 infection in treatment-naive patients based on phase 3 clinical trials, ION-1 and ION-3. In the former, 865 treatment-naive patients with cirrhosis were included, and the latter recruited 647 treatment-naive patients, which excluded people with cirrhosis [26, 27]. In ION-1, SVR12 was 97% to 99% across all study arms with no difference in SVR based on length of treatment, use of ribavirin, or genotype 1 subtype [26]. ION-3 investigated treatment duration for 8 weeks and was found that it was still effective for HCV genotype 1 infection without cirrhosis (SVR 94%), and no further benefit was found by adding ribavirin (SVR 93%). Adverse events included fatigue, nausea, and headache, and there was a higher incidence of these events on the cohort receiving ribavirin, along with the presence of anemia, cough, pruritus, rash, insomnia, and irritability [27, 28].

Table 2. Showing recommended treatment regimens for chronic Hepatitis C based on genotypes

Genotype
Genotype 1 Patients Without Cirrhosis
Daily fixed-dose combination of ledipasvir (90 mg)/sofosbuvir (400 mg)
Daily fixed-dose combination of ledipasvir (90 mg)/sofosbuvir (400 mg) for patients who are non-black, HIV-uninfected, and whose HCV RNA level is <6 million IU/Ml (genotype 1a)*
Daily fixed-dose combination of sofosbuvir (400 mg)/velpatasvir (100 mg)
Genotype 2 Patients Without Cirrhosis
Daily fixed-dose combination of sofosbuvir (400 mg)/velpatasvir (100 mg)
Genotype 4 Patients Without Cirrhosis
Daily fixed-dose combination of sofosbuvir (400 mg)/velpatasvir (100 mg)
Daily fixed-dose combination of ledipasvir (90 mg)/sofosbuvir (400 mg)
Genotype 5 or 6 Patients
Daily fixed-dose combination of sofosbuvir (400 mg)/velpatasvir (100 mg)
Daily fixed-dose combination of ledipasvir (90 mg)/sofosbuvir (400 mg)
Daily fixed-dose combination of sofosbuvir (400 mg)/velpatasvir (100 mg)/voxilaprevir (100 mg) DAA-Experienced (Including NS5A Inhibitors)

Source: Hepatitis C Guidance 2018 Update: AASLD-IDSA Recommendations for Testing, Managing, and Treating Hepatitis C Virus Infection.

Note: * 8 Weeks treatment duration, all other regimens are given daily for 12 weeks.

7.1.2. Sofosbuvir/Velpatasvir

The fixed-dose combination of 12 weeks of sofosbuvir (400 mg)/velpatasvir (100 mg) was approved by the FDA for the treatment of genotype 1 infection in treatment-naive patients based on ASTRAL-1 clinical trials. This placebo-controlled trial involved a 12-week course of sofosbuvir/velpatasvir administered to 624 participants with genotype 1, 2, 4, 5, or 6 who were treatment-naive (n = 423) or previously treated with interferon-based therapy, with or without ribavirin or a protease inhibitor (n = 201) [29]. Of the 328 genotypes 1 patient included, 323 achieved SVR with no difference observed by subtype (98% 1a; 99% 1b).

The phase 3 POLARIS-2 study randomized 941 DAA-naive patients with genotypes 1, 2, 3, 4, 5, or 6 [30]. Among participants treated with sofosbuvir/velpatasvir, 170/172 (99%) with genotype 1a and 57/59 (97%)

with genotype 1b achieved SVR with only a single relapse observed in each subtype.

In real-world studies, it was highlighted by the study of Gayam, et al. among African–American patients in community-based settings and the study of Pan et al. among Asian-Americans that SVR rates remain consistently high regardless of race, and thus support previously completed clinical trials [17, 31].

7.1.3. Simeprevir + Sofosbuvir

The OPTIMIST-1 trial investigated the safety and efficacy of simeprevir (150 mg) and sofosbuvir (400 mg) in patients with genotype 1 without cirrhosis. Overall SVR12 rates were 97% (150/155) for the 12-week arm and 83% (128/155) for the 8-week arm, with a statistically significantly greater relapse rate in the 8-week arm. In terms of safety, frequent adverse events were the same as any DAA regimens, which included nausea, headache, and fatigue. No patients discontinued treatment due to an adverse event [32].

In OPTIMIST-2, patients with HCV genotype 1 with cirrhosis were evaluated for 12 weeks. Of the 103 patients that received treatment, the overall SVR rate was 83%, with treatment naïve patients having a higher SVR than treatment-experienced patients (n = 44/50 88% vs. n = 42/53 79%). Although serious adverse events were noted for 5% of the population, none was considered related to study treatment [33].

7.1.4. Daclatasvir + Sofosbuvir

The phase 3 ALLY-2 trial assessed the efficacy and safety of daclatasvir (60 mg) plus sofosbuvir (400 mg) for the treatment of genotype 1 infection for 12 weeks in patients co-infected with Human Immunodeficiency Virus (HIV) and HCV genotypes 1, 2, 3, or 4 [34]. Among 203 patients enrolled in the study, 123 patients (83%) receiving 12 weeks of therapy in the trial were infected with genotype 1. Eighty-three (54%) of these patients were treatment-naive. SVR rate for genotype 1 patients was 96.4% for patients treated with 12 weeks and 75.6% for those who received 8 weeks of treatment. Common adverse events noted were fatigue, headache, and nausea [34].

It is of particular note that caution should be advised when treating the patient in HCV/HIV co-infected groups. In a real-world community setting, a study conducted by *Gayam* et al. revealed that SVR rates were lower among patients with HCV/HIV co-infection vs. those with mono-infection (84% vs. 94%) [35]. Regardless of efficacy, the safety of sofosbuvir-based DAA regimens remains to be high, as there was no patient who discontinued treatment due to adverse effects (most common was fatigue).

In the ALLY-1 clinical trial, patients with advanced cirrhosis or post-liver transplantation were recruited and given daclatasvir and sofosbuvir. Seventy-six percent of patients enrolled were genotype 1. In patients with cirrhosis, 82% achieved SVR; it was noted that patients with Child-Pugh A or B had a higher SVR rate when compared to those with Child-Pugh C (93% vs. 56%) [36]. This suggests that advancing liver cirrhosis affects overall treatment response, but it is still recommended as the treatment of choice for these populations because of a good safety profile and higher efficacy than previous IFN-based regimens [36]. Post-transplant patients achieved a high SVR rate as well regardless of this co-morbidity (95% SVR rate).

7.2. HCV Genotype 2

7.2.1. Daclatasvir + Sofosbuvir

A prospective study conducted by Mangia et al. observed genotype 2 patients who are either treatment-experienced with contraindication to the use of ribavirin or treatment naïve. One hundred six patients were enrolled and given daclatasvir (60mg) plus sofosbuvir (400mg) once daily for 12 or 24 weeks. Majority of the patients had cirrhosis (58%) and were treatment-experienced (58%), regardless of treatment duration, all patients achieved SVR, and none discontinuation of treatment was observed due to adverse events [37].

7.2.2. Sofosbuvir/Velpatasvir

The POLARIS-2 phase 3 study randomized DAA-naive patients to 8 weeks of sofosbuvir (400 mg)/velpatasvir (100 mg)/voxilaprevir (100mg) versus 12 weeks of sofosbuvir/velpatasvir. Fifty-three patients with genotype 2 were included in the sofosbuvir/velpatasvir arm, and 98% achieved SVR. The study showed that sofosbuvir/velpatasvir/voxilaprevir was not non-inferior to sofosbuvir/velpatasvir and that high efficacy and safety can be achieved with this DAA regimen [30].

7.3. HCV Genotype 3

7.3.1. Sofosbuvir/Velpatasvir

The daily fixed-dose combination of sofosbuvir (400 mg)/velpatasvir (100 mg) for 12 weeks is recommended by the AASLD-IDSA for the treatment of genotype 3 infections in patients without cirrhosis or with compensated cirrhosis [16]. In ASTRAL-3, 552 HCV genotype 3 patients began treatment, 277 patients received sofosbuvir/velpatasvir for 12 weeks, and 275 patients received sofosbuvir plus ribavirin for 24 weeks. SVR rate for the sofosbuvir/velpatasvir group was 95%, which was significantly higher than the 80% SVR rate of the sofosbuvir plus ribavirin group [38].

In POLARIS-3, patients with genotype 3 and cirrhosis were recruited and given sofosbuvir/velpatasvir, and sofosbuvir/velpatasvir/voxilaprevir fixed-dose combinations and was compared to a performance goal of 83%. Results yielded a statistically significant result; 96% of patients achieved SVR12 in both treatment groups, which was higher than the performance goal. Furthermore, the regimen was well tolerated, with a discontinuation rate range of 0 - 1% [30]. Both regimens are, therefore recommended by the AASLD in the treatment of HCV genotype 3 infections [16].

7.3.2. Daclatasvir + Sofosbuvir

ALLY-3 investigated daclatasvir (60 mg) plus sofosbuvir (400 mg) for 12 weeks in patients with HCV genotype 3 infection, treatment naïve, or treatment-experienced patients [39]. SVR rates for both were high (91/101

90% vs. 44/51 86%), and patients without cirrhosis achieved higher SVR rates when compared to those with cirrhosis (105/109 96% vs. 20/32 63%). As with all DAA regimens, the safety tolerability profiles remain excellent, with only 1 treatment discontinuation due to a non-related incident [39].

7.4. HCV Genotype 4

7.4.1. Sofosbuvir/Velpatasvir

The daily fixed-dose combination of sofosbuvir (400 mg)/velpatasvir (100 mg) for 12 weeks was approved by the FDA for the treatment of genotype 4 infections in patients with or without cirrhosis. ASTRAL-1 included 116 genotypes 4-infected treated with sofosbuvir/velpatasvir and 22 patients treated with placebo. All the patients achieved SVR [29].

The POLARIS-2 phase 3 study randomized DAA-naive patients to 8 weeks of sofosbuvir (400 mg)/velpatasvir (100 mg)/voxilaprevir (100 mg) versus 12 weeks of sofosbuvir/velpatasvir. Of the 57 patients with genotype 4 in the sofosbuvir/velpatasvir arm, 98% achieved SVR, and 1 patient experienced relapse [30].

In the real-world study conducted by *Gayam* et al., 100% of patients achieved SVR 12 for those patients who have HCV Genotype 4 Infection in the community setting. The patient was primarily Egyptian descent population [40].

7.4.2. Ledipasvir/Sofosbuvir

The SYNERGY trial was an open-label study which evaluated 12 weeks of ledipasvir (90 mg)/sofosbuvir (400 mg) in 21 HCV genotype 4 infected patients, of whom 60% were treatment-naive, and 43% had advanced fibrosis (Metavir stage F3 or F4) [41]. SVR rate was 95% using intention-to-treat analysis for the cohort (1 withdrew from the study), which included 7 patients having cirrhosis. Again, no discontinuations of treatment were observed, and the treatment was well tolerated. Limitations of this study include a small sample size, which may necessitate further research to adequately represent the general population.

7.5. HCV Genotypes 5 or 6

7.5.1. Sofosbuvir/Velpatasvir
The daily fixed-dose combination of sofosbuvir (400 mg)/velpatasvir (100 mg) for 12 weeks was approved by the FDA for the treatment of genotype 5 and 6 infections in patients with and without cirrhosis [29]. Thirty-five patients with HCV genotype 5 and 41 patients with genotype 6 achieved high SVR rates (34/35 95% and 41/41 100%).

7.5.2. Ledipasvir/Sofosbuvir
Although there are limited data on patients with genotype 5 infection, the *in vitro* activity of sofosbuvir and ledipasvir are quite good with EC_{50} of 15 nM and 0.081 nM, respectively [42]. Abergel and colleagues conducted a phase 2 trial and reported an overall SVR12 rate of 39/41 95% among patients with genotype 5. Among patients who were treatment-naïve, 20/21 95% achieved SVR, and 8/41 with cirrhosis achieved 89% [43].

8. ASSOCIATION OF HCV AND VITAMIN D LEVELS

Vitamin D deficiency is commonly observed among patients with chronic liver disease, with nearly one-third of these patients having severe vitamin D deficiency (< 12 ng/mL) [44]. Petta et al. retrospectively analyzed the relationship of vitamin D levels with peg-IFN/ribavirin for hepatitis C and reported an association between lower vitamin D serum levels and failure to achieve SVR 12 [45]. This is in contrast to the study conducted by Gayam et al. in the real world, where evidence revealed that treatment involving newer DAA therapy does not influence in achieving SVR 12 in vitamin D deficient patients. Further studies are warranted to evaluate optimal vitamin D levels in patients with cirrhosis [46]. Larger randomized trials are necessary to derive more robust conclusions.

Conclusion

In the last few years, a paradigm change in the development of HCV therapeutic regimens has emerged. Because of the high safety, tolerability, and ease of use of DAAs, compliance, and treatment response have been improved on all patients regardless of genotype, race, or treatment status.

Several clinical trials have successfully revealed that sofosbuvir in combination with other DAA resulted in higher SVR 12 in treatment-naive as well as treatment-experienced patients across all HCV genotypes. Due to these reasons, sofosbuvir-containing regimens are highly recommended as the first-line treatment for HCV, even in diverse populations.

References

[1] Buckley, GJ; Strom, BL. A national strategy for the elimination of viral hepatitis emphasizes prevention, screening, and universal treatment of hepatitis C. *Annals of internal medicine.*, 2017, 166(12), 895-6.

[2] Lozano, R; Naghavi, M; Foreman, K; Lim, S; Shibuya, K; Aboyans, V; et al. Global and regional mortality from 235 causes of death for 20 age groups in 1990 and 2010: a systematic analysis for the Global Burden of Disease Study 2010. *The lancet*, 2012, 380(9859), 2095-128.

[3] Freeman, AJ; Dore, GJ; Law, MG; Thorpe, M; Von Overbeck, J; Lloyd, AR; et al. Estimating progression to cirrhosis in chronic hepatitis C virus infection. *Hepatology*, 2001, 34(4), 809-16.

[4] Morgan, RL; Baack, B; Smith, BD; Yartel, A; Pitasi, M; Falck-Ytter, Y. Eradication of hepatitis C virus infection and the development of hepatocellular carcinoma: a meta-analysis of observational studies. *Annals of internal medicine.*, 2013, 158(5_Part_1), 329-37.

[5] Butt, AA; Wang, X; Moore, CG. Effect of hepatitis C virus and its treatment on survival. *Hepatology*, 2009, 50(2), 387-92.

[6] Ghany, MG; Nelson, DR; Strader, DB; Thomas, DL; Seeff, LB. An update on treatment of genotype 1 chronic hepatitis C virus infection: 2011 practice guideline by the American Association for the Study of Liver Diseases. *Hepatology*, 2011, 54(4), 1433-44.

[7] Butt, AA; Kanwal, F. Boceprevir and telaprevir in the management of hepatitis C virus–infected patients. *Clinical infectious diseases.*, 2011, 54(1), 96-104.

[8] Gentile, I; Borgia, F; Buonomo, R; Castaldo, A; Borgia, GG. A novel promising therapeutic option against hepatitis C virus: an oral nucleotide NS5B polymerase inhibitor sofosbuvir. *Current medicinal chemistry*, 2013, 20(30), 3733-42.

[9] Gentile, I; Borgia, F; Zappulo, E; Riccardo Buonomo, A; Maria, Spera A; Castaldo, G; et al. Efficacy and safety of sofosbuvir in the treatment of chronic hepatitis C: the dawn of a new era. *Reviews on recent clinical trials.*, 2014, 9(1), 1-7.

[10] Chen, SL; Morgan, TR. The natural history of hepatitis C virus (HCV) infection. *Int J Med Sci.*, 2006, 3(2), 47-52.

[11] Ryder, SD; Beckingham, IJ. ABC of diseases of liver, pancreas, and biliary system: Acute hepatitis. *BMJ*, 2001, 322(7279), 151-3.

[12] Williams, I; Sabin, K; Fleenor, M; Judson, F; Mottram, K; Poujade, J; et al., editors. Current patterns of hepatitis C virus transmission in the United States. The role of drugs and sex. *Hepatology*; 1998: WB Saunders Co Independence Square West Curtis Center, Ste 300, Philadelphia....

[13] Orland, JR; Wright, TL; Cooper, S. Acute hepatitis C. *Hepatology.*, 2001, 33(2), 321-7.

[14] Seeff, LB. Natural history of chronic hepatitis C. *Hepatology*, 2002, 36(5B), s35-s46.

[15] Lingala, S; Ghany, MG. Natural history of hepatitis C. *Gastroenterology Clinics.*, 2015, 44(4), 717-34.

[16] Panel A-IHG. Hepatitis C Guidance 2018 Update: AASLD-IDSA Recommendations for Testing, Managing, and Treating Hepatitis C Virus Infection. *Clin Infect Dis.*, 2018, 67(10), 1477-92.

[17] Gayam, V; Tiongson, B; Khalid, M; Mandal, AK; Mukhtar, O; Gill, A; et al. Sofosbuvir based regimens in the treatment of chronic hepatitis C genotype 1 infection in African–American patients: a community-based retrospective cohort study. *European journal of gastroenterology & hepatology*, 2018, 30(10), 1200.

[18] Poynard, T; McHutchison, J; Manns, M; Trepo, C; Lindsay, K; Goodman, Z; et al. Impact of pegylated interferon alfa-2b and ribavirin on liver fibrosis in patients with chronic hepatitis C. *Gastroenterology.*, 2002, 122(5), 1303-13.

[19] Morgan, RL; Baack, B; Smith, BD; Yartel, A; Pitasi, M; Falck-Ytter, Y. Eradication of hepatitis C virus infection and the development of hepatocellular carcinoma: a meta-analysis of observational studies. *Ann Intern Med.*, 2013, 158(5 Pt 1), 329-37.

[20] Gisbert, JP; Garcia-Buey, L; Pajares, JM; Moreno-Otero, R. Systematic review: regression of lymphoproliferative disorders after treatment for hepatitis C infection. *Aliment Pharmacol Ther.*, 2005, 21(6), 653-62.

[21] Takahashi, K; Nishida, N; Kawabata, H; Haga, H; Chiba, T. Regression of Hodgkin lymphoma in response to antiviral therapy for hepatitis C virus infection. *Intern Med.*, 2012, 51(19), 2745-7.

[22] van der Meer, AJ; Veldt, BJ; Feld, JJ; Wedemeyer, H; Dufour, JF; Lammert, F; et al. Association between sustained virological response and all-cause mortality among patients with chronic hepatitis C and advanced hepatic fibrosis. *JAMA*, 2012, 308(24), 2584-93.

[23] Boscarino, JA; Lu, M; Moorman, AC; Gordon, SC; Rupp, LB; Spradling, PR; et al. Predictors of poor mental and physical health status among patients with chronic hepatitis C infection: the Chronic Hepatitis Cohort Study (CHeCS). *Hepatology*, 2015, 61(3), 802-11.

[24] Cholongitas, E; Papatheodoridis, GV. Sofosbuvir: a novel oral agent for chronic hepatitis C. *Annals of Gastroenterology: Quarterly Publication of the Hellenic Society of Gastroenterology.*, 2014, 27(4), 331.

[25] Keating, GM; Vaidya, A. Sofosbuvir: first global approval. *Drugs*, 2014, 74(2), 273-82.
[26] Afdhal, N; Zeuzem, S; Kwo, P; Chojkier, M; Gitlin, N; Puoti, M; et al. Ledipasvir and sofosbuvir for untreated HCV genotype 1 infection. *N Engl J Med.*, 2014, 370(20), 1889-98.
[27] Kowdley, KV; Gordon, SC; Reddy, KR; Rossaro, L; Bernstein, DE; Lawitz, E; et al. Ledipasvir and sofosbuvir for 8 or 12 weeks for chronic HCV without cirrhosis. *N Engl J Med.*, 2014, 370(20), 1879-88.
[28] Kowdley, KV; Lawitz, E; Crespo, I; Hassanein, T; Davis, MN; DeMicco, M; et al. Sofosbuvir with pegylated interferon alfa-2a and ribavirin for treatment-naive patients with hepatitis C genotype-1 infection (ATOMIC): an open-label, randomised, multicentre phase 2 trial. *The Lancet*, 2013, 381(9883), 2100-7.
[29] Feld, JJ; Jacobson, IM; Hézode, C; Asselah, T; Ruane, PJ; Gruener, N; et al. Sofosbuvir and velpatasvir for HCV genotype 1, 2, 4, 5, and 6 infection. *New England Journal of Medicine*, 2015, 373(27), 2599-607.
[30] Jacobson, IM; Lawitz, E; Gane, EJ; Willems, BE; Ruane, PJ; Nahass, RG; et al. Efficacy of 8 weeks of sofosbuvir, velpatasvir, and voxilaprevir in patients with chronic HCV infection: 2 phase 3 randomized trials. *Gastroenterology*, 2017, 153(1), 113-22.
[31] Pan, CQ; Tiongson, BC; Hu, KQ; Han, SB; Tong, M; Chu, D; et al. Real-World Study on Sofosbuvir-based Therapies in Asian Americans With Chronic Hepatitis C. *J Clin Gastroenterol.*, 2019, 53(2), 147-54.
[32] Kwo, P; Gitlin, N; Nahass, R; Bernstein, D; Etzkorn, K; Rojter, S; et al. Simeprevir plus sofosbuvir (12 and 8 weeks) in hepatitis C virus genotype 1-infected patients without cirrhosis: OPTIMIST-1, a phase 3, randomized study. *Hepatology*, 2016, 64(2), 370-80.
[33] Lawitz, E; Matusow, G; DeJesus, E; Yoshida, EM; Felizarta, F; Ghalib, R; et al. Simeprevir plus sofosbuvir in patients with chronic hepatitis C virus genotype 1 infection and cirrhosis: A phase 3 study (OPTIMIST-2). *Hepatology*, 2016, 64(2), 360-9.

[34] Wyles, DL; Ruane, PJ; Sulkowski, MS; Dieterich, D; Luetkemeyer, A; Morgan, TR; et al. Daclatasvir plus sofosbuvir for HCV in patients coinfected with HIV-1. *New England Journal of Medicine,* 2015, 373(8), 714-25.

[35] Gayam, V; Hossain, MR; Khalid, M; Chakaraborty, S; Mukhtar, O; Dahal, S; et al. Real-world clinical efficacy and tolerability of direct-acting antivirals in hepatitis C monoinfection compared to hepatitis C/human immunodeficiency virus coinfection in a community care setting. *Gut and liver,* 2018, 12(6), 694.

[36] Poordad, F; Schiff, ER; Vierling, JM; Landis, C; Fontana, RJ; Yang, R; et al. Daclatasvir with sofosbuvir and ribavirin for hepatitis C virus infection with advanced cirrhosis or post-liver transplantation recurrence. *Hepatology,* 2016, 63(5), 1493-505.

[37] Mangia, A; Arleo, A; Copetti, M; Miscio, M; Piazzolla, V; Santoro, R; et al. The combination of daclatasvir and sofosbuvir for curing genotype 2 patients who cannot tolerate ribavirin. *Liver Int.,* 2016, 36(7), 971-6.

[38] Foster, GR; Afdhal, N; Roberts, SK; Bräu, N; Gane, EJ; Pianko, S; et al. Sofosbuvir and velpatasvir for HCV genotype 2 and 3 infection. *New England Journal of Medicine,* 2015, 373(27), 2608-17.

[39] Nelson, DR; Cooper, JN; Lalezari, JP; Lawitz, E; Pockros, PJ; Gitlin, N; et al. All-oral 12-week treatment with daclatasvir plus sofosbuvir in patients with hepatitis C virus genotype 3 infection: ALLY-3 phase III study. *Hepatology,* 2015, 61(4), 1127-35.

[40] Gayam, V; Khalid, M; Mandal, AK; Hussain, MR; Mukhtar, O; Gill, A; et al. Direct-Acting Antivirals in Chronic Hepatitis C Genotype 4 Infection in Community Care Setting. *Gastroenterology research,* 2018, 11(2), 130.

[41] Kohli, A; Kapoor, R; Sims, Z; Nelson, A; Sidharthan, S; Lam, B; et al. Ledipasvir and sofosbuvir for hepatitis C genotype 4: a proof-of-concept, single-centre, open-label phase 2a cohort study. *The Lancet Infectious Diseases,* 2015, 15(9), 1049-54.

[42] Wong, KA; Worth, A; Martin, R; Svarovskaia, E; Brainard, DM; Lawitz, E; et al. Characterization of hepatitis C virus resistance from

a multiple-dose clinical trial of the novel NS5A inhibitor GS-5885. *Antimicrobial agents and chemotherapy.*, 2013, 57(12), 6333-40.

[43] Abergel, A; Asselah, T; Metivier, S; Kersey, K; Jiang, D; Mo, H; et al. Ledipasvir-sofosbuvir in patients with hepatitis C virus genotype 5 infection: an open-label, multicentre, single-arm, phase 2 study. *The Lancet infectious diseases.*, 2016, 16(4), 459-64.

[44] Arteh, J; Narra, S; Nair, S. Prevalence of vitamin D deficiency in chronic liver disease. *Digestive diseases and sciences,* 2010, 55(9), 2624-8.

[45] Petta, S; Cammà, C; Scazzone, C; Tripodo, C; Di Marco, V; Bono, A; et al. Low vitamin D serum level is related to severe fibrosis and low responsiveness to interferon-based therapy in genotype 1 chronic hepatitis C. *Hepatology.*, 2010, 51(4), 1158-67.

[46] Gayam, V; Mandal, AK; Khalid, M; Mukhtar, O; Gill, A; Garlapati, P; et al. Association between Vitamin D Levels and Treatment Response to Direct-Acting Antivirals in Chronic Hepatitis C: A Real-World Study. *Gastroenterology research,* 2018, 11(4), 309.

In: The Pharmacological Guide to Sofosbuvir   ISBN: 978-1-53616-476-3
Editor: Vijay Gayam   © 2019 Nova Science Publishers, Inc.

Chapter 3

INITIAL MANAGEMENT OPTIONS INVOLVING SOFOSBUVIR IN CHRONIC HEPATITIS C INFECTION WITH LIVER CIRRHOSIS

Vijay Gayam[1,*], *MD, Arshpal Gill*[2,†], *MD, Ricky Lali*[3,‡], *Pavani Garlapati*[1,§], *MD, Eric O. Then*[4,∥], *MD, Srikanth Maddika*[4,¶], *MD and Vinaya Gaduputi*[4,#], *MD*

[1]Department of Internal Medicine, Interfaith Medical Center, Brooklyn, NY, US
[2]American University of Antigua, Osbourn, Antigua & Barbuda
[3]Department of Pathology and Molecular Medicine, McMaster University, Hamilton, ON, Canada
[4]Internal Medicine, St. Barnabas Hospital Health System, Bronx, US

---

* Corresponding Author's E-mail: vgayam@interfaithmedical.org.
† Author's E-mail: arshgillmd@gmail.com.
‡ Author's E-mail: alir@mcmaster.ca.
§ Author's E-mail: docpavanireddy@gmail.com.
∥ Author's E-mail: Ericomarthen27@yahoo.com.
¶ Author's E-mail: smaddika@sbhny.org.
# Author's E-mail: Vgaduputi@sbhny.org.

ABSTRACT

Hepatitis C Virus (HCV) is a blood-borne pathogen that afflicts millions around the world. It initially results in acute infection but can become chronic. As a chronic infection, it can lead to the development of compensated cirrhosis, decompensated cirrhosis, necessitation for liver transplantation, and hepatocellular carcinoma. Treatment historically was difficult, as interferon-based regimens were minimally effective and had numerous side effects.

Further complicating treatment is the various genotypes observed in HCV. The error-prone polymerase of HCV results in unique sub-viruses, which have their properties and geographic prevalence. It was essential to public health policymakers and clinicians to establish a safe and effective treatment for Hepatitis C across all genotypes.

Additionally, the chronic nature of the virus means that many patients have already developed compensated and decompensated cirrhosis, so a truly effective HCV treatment must be effective in the later stages of the natural history of HCV infection. Fortunately, it appears the relatively novel concept of direct-acting antivirals (DAA) provides clinicians with a solution. DAA treatments are effective and well-tolerated. Sofosbuvir is a nucleoside analog which helped usher in the era of DAA. In particular, Sofosbuvir is also one half of a regimen which may be considered pan-genotypic. This chapter looks at the effectiveness of direct-acting antiviral regimens which involve sofosbuvir in patients who have already developed cirrhosis.

Keywords: sofosbuvir, Hepatitis C, direct-acting anti-virals, cirrhosis

ABBREVIATIONS

DAA   Direct-acting anti-virals
HAART   Highly Active Anti-Retroviral Therapy
HCV   Hepatitis C Virus
SVR   Sustained Virologic Response

WHAT IS HEPATITIS C?

Hepatitis C Virus (HCV) is a blood-borne pathogen which may result in chronic infection. A chronic HCV infection carries a high burden of disease, as it is one of the most common causes of severe hepatic pathologies which include hepatic fibrosis, hepatic cirrhosis, and hepatocellular carcinoma [1, 2].

The opioid crisis in low income and medically underserved areas have exacerbated many concerns about HCV. Needle sharing amongst infectious hosts and susceptible populations is a cause of an increased incidence in new HCV infections. The current global prevalence of HCV is estimated to have risen from 2.3% to 2.8% over the past decade [3]. An alarming figure with the increased incidence is that lower-resource regions (e.g., India, East Asia, and North Africa) are contributing to the majority of the global burden (~80%) [2, 4]. A lower resource region would likely face more difficulties in addressing HCV as a public health concern.

Due to the infectious and chronic nature of this pathology, there is a strong rationale to institute a robust standard of care treatment that is both accessible and efficacious. Previously, interferon-based regimens were the standard of care for HCV infections [1]. They were minimally effective and had multiple side effects, including fatigue and anemia. This is problematic for the patient, but also policymakers as severe symptoms will often decrease adherence to treatment, thus contributing to treatment failure [5].

Fortunately, the recent development of direct-acting antiviral (DAA) regimens, many of which include sofosbuvir, provides clinicians with a safer and more effective treatment when combating HCV. Their effectiveness will be discussed in this chapter. The use of interferon and ribavirin-free regimens are associated with higher adherence and are more effective [1, 5]. This provides clinicians and public health policy officials with the optimism that not only can we treat existing patients with HCV but also mitigate the existence of the current infectious reservoir.

The existence of DAA regimens is a relatively novel concept, and due to the previous treatment in interferon-based regimens being less than effective, many patients have already developed compensated cirrhosis [1, 6]. The natural history of HCV involves an acute infection which will become chronic in certain individuals. The acute phase may be clinically silent, making the possibility of an early diagnosis more challenging. The progression of the disease is often slow and involves a gradual progression from fibrosis to cirrhosis with an increased incidence of hepatocellular carcinoma [1, 7]. Additionally, many patients will have advanced pathology due to the silent nature of the disease and may only be noticed in the cirrhotic stages [8]. As such, it is important to have a therapy that is effective and safe in patients with compensated cirrhosis. Initial studies involving Sofosbuvir and ribavirin showed that the presence of cirrhosis was a hindrance in achieving a successful sustained virologic response (SVR) [9]. Worsening of compensated cirrhosis into decompensation, or the necessitation for a liver transplant are undesirable patient outcomes.

Indeed, the current annual risk for development of hepatic decompensation and hepatocellular carcinoma among patients with cirrhosis is 5-7% and 1-5%, respectively (among all genotypes) [4, 6, 10]. Moreover, HCV-associated hepatic cirrhosis remains among the foremost causes of end-stage liver disease requiring transplantation. Well powered population studies have shown that age among individuals with hepatic cirrhosis confers a 3% increase risk in waitlist mortality per year [11], thus establishing the need for robust therapeutic intervention at the time of diagnosis across all HCV genotypes to prevent the accumulation of unnecessary risk. Additionally, it has been demonstrated that mortality rates among individuals allocated to a low score Model for End-stage Liver Disease Sodium (MLEDNa) groups (i.e., MLEDNa < 15) are grossly underestimated [12]. Since the MLEDNa is the standard gold metric for categorizing urgency of liver transplantation, higher than expected mortality rates among individuals with established hepatic decompensation represents an urgent need to 1) refine liver allocation criteria and 2) institute point of care therapy that results in high viral clearance with limited rates of recurrence. The most common indication for a liver transplant in the United States remains to be HCV related cirrhosis. Liver transplants also represent an extensive cost on healthcare systems [13].

Historically, interferon-based regimens were poorly tolerated in patients with common side effects including fatigue and anemia. The development of direct-acting antivirals represent an interferon-free and ribavirin-free regimen, and the presence of interferon and ribavirin historically meant that patient adherence was lower than desired [5]. Studies conducted involving show that DAA appears to be much more effective and better tolerated than its predecessors [14-17].

An additional factor complicating the treatment of HCV infection involves the process of selecting an appropriate DAA regimen. HCV has a high replication rate and the low fidelity of the RNA-dependent RNA polymerase acting on the positive-sense RNA of HCV results in high genomic mutability [18]. Consequently, there are many demarcated HCV genotypes. Each genotype is characterized by a different prevalence depending on geographic region and each unique exhibit characteristics. Nevertheless, all genotypes demonstrated an inconsistently poor response to traditional pegylated interferon-based treatments, which also came with numerous side effects [14, 15, 17, 19]. The selection of a DAA regimen is usually informed based on the HCV genotype with which the patient has been afflicted. However, specifically about Sofosbuvir, there is the possibility of a pan-genotypic regimen which would eliminate the necessity for genotype testing.

There needs to be an initiative amongst clinicians and public health policymakers to successfully implement DAA regimens (including Sofosbuvir-based treatment regimens) across all HCV genotypes. The current regimens appear effective in compensated hepatic cirrhosis, which is crucial as preventing decompensation and avoiding hepatic transplant should be critical goals when concerning ideal patient outcomes.

WHAT IS SOFOSBUVIR?

Sofosbuvir is a nucleoside analog, which has been approved by the Food and Drug Administration in the treatment of HCV infection. It functions through its ability to inhibit HCV polymerase [17]. Specifically,

Sofosbuvir functions as a nucleoside monophosphate prodrug analog of a uridine residue and are activated by hepatic carboxylesterase 1 and nucleoside kinases to generate into an active triphosphate residue [20, 21]. The activated form of Sofosbuvir acts as an inactive substrate for the NS5B HCV polymerase by preventing nucleotide elongation due to the steric hindrance caused by a 2' methyl group on its ribose ring. In its metabolically active form, Sofosbuvir has a maximal plasma concentration (C-max) of 567 ng/mL that is obtained within 0.5-2 hours, a 24-hour plasma exposure of 8200 ng-h/ml, and a plasma half-life of 27 hours [21]. Additionally, the plasma absorption efficiency of Sofosbuvir is not influenced by diet type as is the case for DAA's acting as protease and NS5A inhibitors, which demonstrate limited absorption among individuals with fatty diets [6]. Other common HCV DAA's are NS3/4A protease and NS5A inhibitors, which collectively participate in processing the HCV polyprotein into active virulence factors that are necessary for viral assembly and replication [22]. However, since these DAA's do not act directly on the polymerase activity, the NS5B polymerase retains residual enzymatic activity and is still able to contribute to the mutability of the HCV RNA genome [23]. As such, NS3/4A protease and NS5A inhibitors have low barriers for viral resistance, which furthers the necessity of extensive combination therapies and potential unfavorable drug-drug interactions. By its mechanism of action, Sofosbuvir has demonstrated a high genetic barrier to resistance with <1% of individuals showing no SVR response throughout all pertinent clinical trials treating HCV mono-infected individuals [14, 15, 17, 24, 25]. Furthermore, Sofosbuvir is not metabolically dependent upon cytochrome P450 (CP450) enzymes and therefore circumvents drug-drug interaction that plague first and second-generation protease and NS5A inhibitors.

Sofosbuvir has an important role in DAA therapy as the AASLD has several approved DAA regimens which involve Sofosbuvir. Sofosbuvir appears to be safe, even in the elderly population which is another important feature [26]. Finally, all indicators point to the fact that Sofosbuvir is a cost-effective drug [27].

Current AASLD guideline approved Sofosbuvir-based regimens include Ledipasvir/Sofosbuvir, Sofosbuvir and Velptasavir, Sofosbuvir/Daclatasvir, and Sofosbuvir/Velptasavir/Voxiplrevir. When concerning the initial treatment of patients with HCV infection and existing compensated cirrhosis, Ledipasvir/Sofosbuvir and Sofosbuvir/ Velpatasvir are mainstays of therapy.

INITIAL AASLD GUIDELINE APPROVED REGIMENS INVOLVING SOFOSBUVIR IN THE TREATMENT OF HEPATITIS C VIRUS PATIENTS WITH EXISTING COMPENSATED CIRRHOSIS

Ledipasvir and Sofosbuvir

Ledipasvir is an inhibitor of the HCV NS5A protein [6]. In conjunction with Sofosbuvir, it creates a DAA regimen which may be used in Genotype 1 infection, Genotype 4 infection, Genotype 5 infection, and Genotype 6 infection [28]. The Ledipasvir/Sofosbuvir combination was examined extensively in the ION-1 trial for Genotype 1 infection, which showed very promising results [17].

Sofosbuvir and Velpatasvir

This is perhaps one of the most promising breakthroughs in DAA regimens. Sofosbuvir/Velpatasvir appears to be effective across all genotypes; a so-called "pan-genotypic" HCV treatment regimen that can standardize care across all HCV-prevalent regions, especially among rarer HCV genotypes (namely, genotype-5 and genotype-6). Moreover, a ubiquitous treatment regimen will preclude health care spending on genotyping assays and will mitigate the misdiagnosis of HCV genotype due to their limitations in sensitivity and specificity. In fact, the ASTRAL-

4 clinical trial demonstrated potential utility of a Sofosbuvir/Velpatasvir direct-acting antiviral (DAA) combination treatment as a potent pangenotypic HCV treatment as it showed a marked increase in SVR 12 weeks after end-of-treatment (i.e., SVR12) for genotypes 1, 2, 4, 5, 6 in patients with decompensated hepatic cirrhosis [29]. Specifically, the SVR12 in patients taking Sofosbuvir/Velpatasivr was 88% and increased to 92% with a 24-week trial. Adding Ribavirin to the Sofosbuvir/Velpatasvir appeared to provide the most effective response in decompensated cirrhosis, as the SVR increased to 96% [29].

The POLARIS-3 trial showed that individuals with genotype 3 and compensated cirrhosis achieved SVR12 of 96% using Sofosbuvir-based combination regimens (Sofosbuvir/Velpatasvir and Sofosbuvir/ Velpatasvir/Voxilaprevir) [25]. The ASTRAL-3 trial also corroborated that Sofosbuvir/Velptasavir has Genotype 3 efficacy [15]. One study which looked at the combined results of ASTRAL-1, ASTRAL-2, ASTRAL-3, and ASTRAL-4 concluded that patient-reported outcomes were greatly improved upon Sofosbuvir/Velpatastvir, including those patients with compensated cirrhosis [30].

Table 1. AASLD Approved DAA Regimens Involving Sofosbuvir for the initial treatment of Hepatitis C in Compensated Cirrhosis [28]

TREATMENT	TREATMENT DURATION
Genotype 1	
Sofosbuvir/Velptasivir	12 weeks
Ledipasvir/Sofosbuvir	12 weeks
Genotype 2	
Sofosbuvir/Velptasivir	12 weeks
Genotype 3	
Sofosbuvir/Velptasivir	12 weeks
Genotype 4	
Sofosbuvir/Velptasivir	12 weeks
Ledipasvir/Sofosbuvir	12 weeks
Genotype 5/6	
Sofosbuvir/Velptasivir	12 weeks
Ledipasvir/Sofosbuvir	12 weeks

SOFOSBUVIR-BASED REGIMENS FOR HCV TREATMENT BY GENOTYPE

Genotype 1 Infection

Of all the various genotype noted in HCV infection, Genotype 1 infection appears to be the most common infection seen globally. Additionally, it is also the most common infection seen in developed countries; which is significant as developed countries are more likely to have the healthcare resources to combat HCV [31]. Combating GT1 infections as early as the fibrotic stages of the natural history of HCV infection have proven cost-effective benefits [32]. There are various regimens involved in the treatment of Genotype 1 infection, but there are two which involve sofosbuvir. Ledipasvir/Sofosbuvir has been heavily studied in the ION trial, while Sofosbuvir/Velpatasvir was examined thoroughly in the ASTRAL-1 trial. Genotype 1 infections are often broken down into Genotype 1a and Genotype1b infections, as illustrated in the ASTRAL-1 trial [33].

Ledipasvir/Sofosbuvir for Genotype 1

The ION-1 study was a clinical trial to assess the efficacy and safety of DAA regimens involving Ledipasvir and Sofosbuvir on Genotype 1 patients [17]. It was hard to determine in the ION-1 trial the exact impact of cirrhosis on efficacy, as the overall SVR remained high. However, the presence of cirrhosis did not change the safety profile. The most common side effects noted in the study included fatigue, headache, nausea, and insomnia [17]. Since Genotype 1 is the most common infection globally, it is important to assess that the Ledipasvir/Sofosbuvir demonstrates real-world efficacy. One real-world study involving patients that were noncirrhotic showed an overall SVR of 96% [34]. Another real-world study involving three different Sofosbuvir regimens for Genotype 1 infection showed an SVR of 93.8% for ledipasvir and Sofosbuvir.

The study included both cirrhotic and non-cirrhotic patients, but the cirrhosis status did not appear to influence SVR [35]. An additional study with nearly half the study population having a Genotype 1 infection and cirrhosis showed an overall high SVR of 96.7% [36]. According to another study, the quality of life also appears to improve with patients taking Ledipasvir/Sofosbuvir in Genotype 1 infections [37]. All these studies help corroborate that Ledipasvir and Sofosbuvir are effective in real-world studies, including in patients with cirrhosis. Ledipasvir/Sofosbuvir also appears to be a cost-effective treatment as well in Genotype 1 infections, particularly when examining patients with existing fibrosis [32].

The typical therapy in patients with no other risk factors for failure including co-infections, African-American race, and cirrhosis, is an 8-week regimen. However, in the presence of cirrhosis, Ledipasvir/Sofosbuvir is recommended for 12 weeks according to the American Association for the Study of Liver Diseases (AASLD) guidelines.

Sofosbuvir/Velpatasvir for Genotype 1

This is a 12-week regimen regardless of cirrhotic status according to the AASLD guidelines, which makes it more unique than L/S where the treatment duration changes with the presence of cirrhosis. The ASTRAL-1 trial examined patients across genotypes 1,2,4,5, and 6, both with and without cirrhosis [14]. Across all genotypes, the ASTRAL-1 study had 19% of the study population's patients being diagnosed with existing cirrhosis. Despite the presence of cirrhosis, the SVR rates were high. Among patients with cirrhosis, 120 out of 121 patients responded to Sofosbuvir/Velpatasvir therapy. There was an SVR of 98% in Genotype 1a infections and a 99% SVR in Genotype 1b infections. This was consistent with the ASTRAL-1 overall study results across all genotypes, which exhibited an overall SVR of 99%. While the ASTRAL-1 study involved 5 out of the six major genotypes, only Genotype 1 exhibited signs of virologic relapse in 2 patients out of the total 624 patients studied [14].

Genotype 2 Infection

Genotype 2 infection is less common than Genotype 1 and Genotype 3 infection, and it is most commonly observed in Eastern Asia [31]. There are several options to consider when compiling an initial treatment plan for Genotype 2 infection; however, there is only one option involving a Sofosbuvir-based regimen; Sofosbuvir/Velpatasvir.

Sofosbuvir/Velpatasvir for Genotype 2
The recommended duration of 12 weeks for Sofosbuvir/Velptasvir appears to be an effective modality to combat Genotype 2 infection as indicated in the ASTRAL-1 study. It remains safe and effective. In Genotype 2 infection patients observed in the ASTRAL-1 study, there was a perfect SVR of 100% in all 104 Genotype 2 patients studied.

The ASTRAL-2 study shows an overall 99% SVR in Genotype patients, including those with cirrhosis, which is higher than the Sofosbuvir/Ribavirin SVR of 94% [15]. Also despite the high presence of resistance strains studied in the Sofosbuvir/Velpatasvir for Genotype 2 population, no virological failures were noted [15]. Nausea, headache, fatigue were common symptoms, and while adverse events, in general, were common, serious adverse events were rare [15], which helps support the tolerability and safety of Sofosbuvir/Velpatasvir in Genotype 2 infections.

Genotype 3 Infection

Genotype 3 infection is most common in South Asia, and after Genotype 1 infection it is the most common infection globally [31]. This is a problem because Genotype 3 infection may be more likely to cause cirrhosis and hepatocellular carcinoma. A national sample indicated that a Genotype 3 infection is more likely to cause cirrhosis than a Genotype 1 infection, which is already considered one of the more aggressive HCV genotypes. In addition to the elevated risk of cirrhosis, Genotype 3 may also be associated with an increased risk in hepatocellular carcinoma, as observed in the same study [38]. Further complicating the problem is that compared to other HCV infections, Genotype 3 infections have a comparatively higher failure rate [39]. One study shows which include Sofosbuvir based regimens and Genotype 3 infections shows promising results, but the presence of cirrhosis still diminishes the response [40]. Therefore, it is important to attempt to target Genotype 3 infections before the development of cirrhosis.

There is currently only 1 approved regimen involving Sofosbuvir for a Genotype 3 infection; which is the Sofosbuvir/Velpatasvir regimen [28].

Sofosbuvir/Velpatasvir for Genotype 3

The ASTRAL-3 study was conducted to see the efficacy and safety of Sofosbuvir/Velpatasvir in Genotype 3 infections. There was a stark difference noted in the presence of cirrhosis, as SVR was 97% in patients without cirrhosis, but only 91% in patients with cirrhosis [15]. Despite the decrease in efficacy, Sofosbuvir/Velpatasvir is still be warranted in Genotype 3 infection as indicated in the AASLD guidelines [28]. The treatment duration for Genotype 3 infection and Sofosbuvir/Velpatasvir is 12 weeks; a duration which doesn't change regardless of whether or not there is cirrhosis. When comparing treatment involving Sofosbuvir and Velpatasvir to Genotype 2 infections, Genotype 3 patients experienced adverse events more frequently [15].

Another study found that adding ribavirin in patients with HCV Genotype 3 infections and existing cirrhosis improved the SVR [41]. The SVR was 91% with just Sofosbuvir/Velpatasvir for Genotype 3, and it increased to 96% with the addition of Ribavirin to the Sofosbuvir/ Velptasvir regimen. However, both figures are acceptably high SVR rates, particularly in the dreaded and difficult to Genotype 3 infection and existing cirrhosis combination.

Lastly, the POLARIS-3 trial enrolled treatment-naïve individuals with Genotype 3 and identified a 96% SVR in treatment groups randomized to either Sofosbuvir/Velpatasvir (at 12 weeks) or Sofosbuvir/Velpatasvir/ Voxilaprevir (at 8 weeks) [25]. The Only 2% of individuals (2/101) in the

Sofosbuvir/Velpatasvir group experienced virological failure that was either due to insufficient HCV-RNA suppression followed by virological rebound or virological relapse [25]. However, due to low concentrations of the primary metabolite of Sofosbuvir, it is likely that cases of virological failure were due to low-adherence to the ascribed treatment regimen. Similarly, only 2% of individuals (2/103) in the Sofosbuvir/Velpatasvir/Voxilaprevir group experienced a virologic relapse [25]. The proportion of adverse side-effects were similar in both groups, except more of nausea and vomiting in the Sofosbuvir/Velpatasvir/Voxilaprevir group [25]. As such Sofosbuvir/Velpatasvir remains a gold-standard regimen for cirrhotic patients afflicted with Genotype 3 to achieve high cure rates while minimizing adverse events.

Genotype 4 Infection

Genotype 4 infections are most commonly seen in North Africa and the Middle East [31]. There are currently two regimens involving Sofosbuvir to treat initial Genotype 4 infection in compensated cirrhosis, Ledipasvir/Sofosbuvir, and Sofosbuvir/Velpatasvir [28].

Ledipasvir/Sofosbuvir for Genotype 4

Ledipasvir/Sofosbuvir appears to be an effective solution in combating Genotype 4 infections. A proof of concept study showed a high SVR of 95% while showing the drug was relatively well-tolerated. Fatigue, diarrhea, nausea, and upper respiratory infection were the most common adverse effects documented [16].

The challenge with Ledipasvir/Sofosbuvir in Genotype 4 infections is the paucity of existing real-world literature. As mentioned earlier, Genotype 4 infections are uncommon globally, and are even more uncommon is higher resource areas which would be able to study Genotype 4 more effectively [31]. One community-based paper showed an overall high SVR of 93.8% in Ledipasvir/Sofosbuvir patients in Genotype

4 infections, but the number dropped drastically when examining patients with compensated cirrhosis, likely due to small sample size [42].

Sofosbuvir/Velpatasvir for Genotype 4

The ASTRAL-1 trial which examined Genotype 1, Genotype 2, Genotype 4, Genotype 5, and Genotype 6 infections had an overall high SVR of 99% [14]. This was also true for Genotype 4 infections, which exhibited an SVR of 100% in the study. The study population included patients with cirrhosis as well, and it appears that cirrhosis wasn't significantly altering the response rate.

Genotype 5 and Genotype 6 Infection

Genotype 5 and Genotype 6 infections are the most uncommon genotype seen in HCV. They have been grouped by the AASLD for treatment infection [28]. Genotype 5 infection is the most uncommon infection of the six major HCV genotypes, and it is most commonly seen in Africa. Genotype 6 infection is most commonly seen in East Asia [31, 43]. Due to the scarcity of Genotype 5 and six outside Northern South Africa and East Asia, respectively, it is difficult for clinical and community-based studies to achieve sufficient statistical power to establish a *bonafide* standard of a care treatment regimen for these genotypes. However, a Sofosbuvir/Velpatasvir combination treatment has been demonstrated promise in achieving high cure rates for Genotype 5 and Genotype 6, albeit among small sample sizes [14]. Therefore, there must be an initiative to identify the efficacy of a Sofosbuvir/Velpatasvir regimen in areas endemic to Genotype 5 and 6 to establish a putative pan-genotypic treatment measure. This would not only preclude health care spending on novel DAA's but would minimize monetary allocation to pegylated interferon-based treatment (with or without ribavirin), which have only demonstrated limited efficacy among both genotypes (31-67% SVR for Genotype 5 [43-47] and 44-88% SVR for Genotype 6 [43, 48-54]).

Ledipasvir/Sofosbuvir for Genotype 5 and Genotype 6

As indicated in the AASLD guidelines Ledipasvir/Sofosbuvir is amongst the recommended treatments for Genotype 5 and Genotype 6 infections. However, there is difficulty in finding enough literature as genotype 5 and six infections are the most uncommon seen. One study showed a Ledipasvir/Sofosbuvir induced SVR of 97% in Genotype 5 patients without cirrhosis. The presence of cirrhosis diminishes the SVR down to 89% [55]. One community-based study examining Ledipasvir/Sofosbuvir on Genotype 6 infections showed an SVR of 97.4% in patients with no cirrhosis, but it diminishes to 92.3% in the presence of cirrhosis [56].

Sofosbuvir/Velpatasvir for Genotype 5 and Genotype 6

Genotype 5 and 6 represents a paucity when comparing more common genotypes. This is also represented in the ASTRAL-1 trial, where there are only 35 Genotype 5 patients, and 41 Genotype 6 patients given Sofosbuvir/Velpatasvir [14]. They both represent the smallest study population by a wide margin in the ASTRAl-1 trial. Genotype 5 was the only study group in ASTRAL-1 which did not undergo randomization due to the scarce nature of the infection [14]. The lack of population size for both Genotype 5 and 6 gave a wider confidence interval; however, the SVR is still promising. Genotype 5 showed a response rate of 97%, and Genotype 6 showed an SVR of 100% [14].

Special Considerations for HCV/HIV Co-Infection

HCV and Human Immunodeficiency Virus (HIV) exhibit similar modes of transmission including through percutaneous exposure to blood, substance abuse, and sexual intercourse. Consequently, HCV-HIV co-infection is common with ~25% of individuals living with HIV also having HCV [57, 58]. However, due to non-systematic screening procedures, it is estimated that >50% and >20% of HCV and HIV cases remain undiagnosed [59]. Unlike HCV mono-infection, HCV-HIV co-infection substantially alters the cellular architecture of the adaptive immune system as both CD4+ T-cells and natural killer (NK) cells become depleted in the co-infected state. Particularly, in the absence of HIV, NK cells can homeostatically modulate the degree of collagen chemo-attraction to hepatocytes through controlling hepatic stem cell apoptosis [59, 60]. Consequently, individuals that are co-infected are at increased risk for hepatic disease progression, including a higher rate of hepatic fibrosis, decompensation, end-stage liver disease, and death [59-61]. Similar to HCV mono-infection, pegylated interferon-based regimens demonstrated poor efficacy (SVR12 < 30%) and tolerance [59-61].

Clinical trials such as ALLY-2 have demonstrated that combination Sofosbuvir-based regimens achieved SVR12 of 92% in co-infected individuals while also minimizing the hepatotoxicity with concomitant Highly Active Anti-Retroviral (HAART) treatment because Sofosbuvir is not metabolized by CP450 enzymes [6, 62]. Furthermore, there have been conflicting results regarding the efficacy of DAA treatment in HCV-HIV co-infection between clinical and real-world study designs. This can largely be attributed to the absence of 1) strict inclusion/exclusion criteria in real-world studies and 2) incentive to remain in a real-world study to its completion. These factors contribute to strong study confounding and less power to detect primary patient outcomes, respectively. Therefore, results obtained from the real-world, community-based studies need to be interpreted with these limiting factors in mind. Real-world studies still show a high SVR in HIV/HCV co-infection when using Sofosbuvir-based regimens [61].

Decompensated Cirrhosis

As established earlier in the chapter, hepatic decompensation is an unfavorable outcome in HCV infection. Patients with HCV with no cirrhosis, or even compensated cirrhosis should undergo immediate DAA selection that is appropriated by the AASLD. One study showed that there is 1-year mortality of 5.4% in compensated cirrhosis, but this figure greatly increases to 20.2% in the presence of decompensated cirrhosis [63].

The ASTRAL-4 study sought out to examine the response rate of Sofosbuvir/Velpatasvir for 12 weeks, Sofosbuvir/Velpatasvir plus ribavirin for 12 weeks, and Sofosbuvir/Velpatasvir for 24 weeks [29]. The scarcity of genotype 5 meant that it was not included in the study. The response rate, defined as SVR, for the 12-week Sofosbuvir/Velpatasvir regimen was observed to be 83%. The response rate for Sofosbuvir/Velpatasvir, when given for 24 weeks in decompensated cirrhosis, increased slightly to 86%. While both figures are lower than the studied conducted in patients with compensated cirrhosis, they still represent a fairly successful therapy given the end-stage nature of decompensated cirrhosis. However, perhaps the most interesting aspect of the ASTRAL-4 study is the response rate observed in patients taking Sofosbuvir/Velpatasvir, and ribavirin for 12 weeks as they responded at an extremely efficient rate of 94%. That number increases to 96% when just examining Genotype 1 infections, which was earlier in the chapter established as the most prevalent HCV infection [29].

The AASLD guidelines incorporated the success of ribavirin into their guidelines when treating decompensated cirrhosis. According to current guidelines, the existing sofosbuvir-based regimens for compensated cirrhosis are acceptable for decompensated cirrhosis as long as ribavirin is added. Additionally, another Sofosbuvir-based regimen, Daclatasvir, and Sofosbuvir may be used alongside ribavirin in Genotype 1-4 infections [28].

Summary of Sofosbuvir-Based Regimens

The following is only a list of examples of various regimens as published in guidelines by the American Association of Study of Liver Diseases. This list is limited to those regimens that contain Sofosbuvir only and assumed that doses had been adjusted appropriately as per clinical necessity.

Treatment-Naive with Compensated Cirrhosis

Genotype 1a/1b:

- Sofosbuvir (400mg)/ Ledipasvir (90mg) daily for 12 weeks
- Sofosbuvir (400mg)/ Velpatasvir (100mg) daily for 12 weeks

Genotype 2:

- Sofosbuvir (400mg)/ Velpatasvir (100mg) daily for 12 weeks
- Sofosbuvir (400mg) / Daclatasvir (60mg) daily for 16 -24 weeks

Genotype 3: Consider RAS testing

- Without Y93H RAS
- Sofosbuvir (400mg)/ Velpatasvir (100mg) daily for 12 weeks
- Y93H RAS positive
- Sofosbuvir (400mg)/Velpatasvir (100mg)/Voxilaprevir(100mg) for 12 weeks
- Sofosbuvir (400mg)/Daclatasvir (60mg)/weight based Ribavirin for 24 weeks.

Genotype 4/5/6:

- Sofosbuvir (400mg)/ Velpatasvir (100mg) daily for 12 weeks
- Sofosbuvir (400mg)/ Ledipasvir (90mg) daily for 12 weeks.

TREATMENT-EXPERIENCED (PEG IFN/RIBAVIRIN) WITH COMPENSATED CIRRHOSIS

Genotype 1a /1b:

- Sofosbuvir (400mg)/ Velpatasvir (100mg) daily for 12 weeks
- Sofosbuvir (400mg)/ Ledipasvir (90mg)/weight based Ribavirin for 12 weeks

Genotype 2:

- Sofosbuvir (400mg)/ Velpatasvir (100mg) daily for 12 weeks
- Sofosbuvir (400mg) / Daclatasvir (60mg) daily for 16- 24 weeks

Genotype 3:

- Sofobuvir (400mg)/Elbasvir (50mg)/Grazoprevir (100mg) – 12 weeks
- Sofosbuvir (400mg)/ Velpatasvir (100mg)/Voxilaprevir (100mg) – 12 weeks
- Sofosbuvir (400mg)/Velpatasvir (100mg)/ Ribavirin – 12 weeks

Genotype 4:

- Sofosbuvir (400mg)/ Velpatasvir (100mg) daily for 12 weeks
- Sofosbuvir (400mg)/ Ledipasvir (90mg)/weight based Ribavirin for 12 weeks

Genotype 5/6:

- Sofosbuvir (400mg)/ Velpatasvir (100mg) daily for 12 weeks
- Sofosbuvir (400mg)/ Ledipasvir (90mg) daily for 12 weeks

TREATMENT-EXPERIENCED (NS3/PEG IFN/ RIBAVIRIN) WITH COMPENSATED CIRRHOSIS

Genotype 1a/1b:

- Sofosbuvir (400mg)/ Velpatasvir (100mg) daily for 12 weeks
- Sofosbuvir (400mg)/ Ledipasvir (90mg) /Ribavirin for 12 weeks

Genotype 2:

- Sofosbuvir (400mg)/ Velpatasvir (100mg) daily for 12 weeks

Genotype 3:

- Sofosbuvir (400mg)/ Velpatasvir (100mg)/Voxilaprevir (100mg) – 12 weeks

Genotype 4:

- Sofosbuvir (400mg)/ Velpatasvir (100mg)/Voxilaprevir (100mg) – 12 weeks

Genotype 5/6:

- Sofosbuvir (400mg)/ Velpatasvir (100mg)/Voxilaprevir (100mg) – 12 weeks

TREATMENT-EXPERIENCED (NON-NS5A/SOFOSBUVIR) WITH COMPENSATED CIRRHOSIS

Genotype 1a:

- Sofosbuvir (400mg)/ Velpatasvir (100mg)/Voxilaprevir (100mg) – 12 weeks

Genotype 1b:

- Sofosbuvir (400mg)/ Velpatasvir (100mg) daily for 12 weeks

Genotype 2:

- Sofosbuvir (400mg)/ Velpatasvir (100mg) daily for 12 weeks

Genotype 3:

- Sofosbuvir (400mg)/ Velpatasvir (100mg)/Voxilaprevir (100mg) – 12 weeks

Genotype 4:

- Sofosbuvir (400mg)/ Velpatasvir (100mg)/Voxilaprevir (100mg) – 12 weeks

Genotype 5/6:

- Sofosbuvir (400mg)/ Velpatasvir (100mg)/Voxilaprevir (100mg) – 12 weeks

Treatment-Experienced (NS5A Inhibitor) with Compensated Cirrhosis

Genotype 1a/1b:

- Sofosbuvir (400mg)/Velpatasvir (100mg)/Voxilaprevir (100mg) – 12 weeks

Genotype 2:

- Sofosbuvir (400mg)/Velpatasvir (100mg)/Voxilaprevir (100mg) – 12 weeks

Genotype 3:

- Sofosbuvir (400mg)/Velpatasvir (100mg)/Voxilaprevir (100mg)/ Ribavirin – 12 weeks

Genotype 4:

- Sofosbuvir (400mg)/Velpatasvir (100mg)/Voxilaprevir (100mg) – 12 weeks

Genotype 5/6:

- Sofosbuvir (400mg)/ Velpatasvir (100mg)/Voxilaprevir (100mg) – 12 weeks.

PATIENTS WITH DECOMPENSATED CIRRHOSIS

Treatment Naïve Patients with Decompensated Cirrhosis / Genotype 1/4/5/6
Ribavirin eligible:

- Sofosbuvir (400mg) / Ledipasvir (90mg) /Ribavirin (start at low dose) – 12 weeks
- Sofosbuvir (400mg) / Velpatasvir (100mg) / Ribavirin – 12 weeks

Ribavirin Ineligible:

- Sofosbuvir (400mg) / Ledipasvir (90mg) - 24 weeks
- Sofosbuvir (400mg) / Velpatasvir (100mg) - 24 weeks

Treatment-Experienced Patients with Decompensated Cirrhosis / Genotype 1/4/5/6

- Sofosbuvir (400mg) / Velpatasvir (100mg) / Ribavirin – 24 weeks

Treatment Naïve Patients with Decompensated cirrhosis / Genotype 2/3

Ribavirin Eligible:

- Sofosbuvir (400mg) / Velpatasvir (100mg) / Ribavirin – 12 weeks
- Sofosbuvir (400mg) / Daclatsvir (60mg) / Ribavirin (start @ low dose) – 12 weeks

Ribavirin Ineligible:

- Sofosbuvir (400mg) / Velpatasvir (100mg) - 24 weeks
- Sofosbuvir (400mg) / Daclatsvir (60mg) – 24 weeks

Treatment-Experienced Patients with Decompensated Cirrhosis / Genotype 2/3

- Sofosbuvir (400mg) / Velpatasvir (100mg) / Ribavirin – 24 weeks

CONCLUSION

Sofosbuvir plays an integral role in the treatment of HCV. It participates in numerous DAA regimens, and as a class of drugs, DAA therapy represents a vastly more effective and well-tolerated treatment when compared to its predecessor in interferon-based regimens. Furthermore, Sofosbuvir-based regimens demonstrated success even in the presence of both compensated cirrhosis and decompensated cirrhosis. This is a desirable property in an HCV therapy, as many patients have already developed advanced hepatic pathology due to the chronic nature of HCV. The cost-effectiveness and the possibility of a pan-genotypic Sofosbuvir based regimen provide clinicians and public health policymakers an effective tool in combating the high burden of disease that is associated with HCV.

REFERENCES

[1] Manns MP, Buti M, Gane E, et al. Hepatitis C virus infection. *Nat Rev Dis Prim*. 2017;3:17006. doi:10.1038/nrdp.2017.6.

[2] Kumar A, Chhabra R, Yadav A, Singh S, Paliwal D, Rajput M. Genotyping & diagnostic methods for hepatitis C virus: A need of low-resource countries. *Indian J Med Res*. 2018;147(5):445. doi:10.4103/ijmr.ijmr_1850_16.

[3] Mohd Hanafiah K, Groeger J, Flaxman AD, Wiersma ST. Global epidemiology of hepatitis C virus infection: New estimates of age-specific antibody to HCV seroprevalence. *Hepatology*. 2013;57(4):1333-1342. doi:10.1002/hep.26141.

[4] Petruzziello A, Marigliano S, Loquercio G, Cozzolino A, Cacciapuoti C. Global epidemiology of hepatitis C virus infection: An up-date of the distribution and circulation of hepatitis C virus genotypes. *World J Gastroenterol*. 2016;22(34):7824-7840. doi:10.3748/wjg.v22.i34.7824.

[5] Younossi ZM, Stepanova M, Henry L, Nader F, Younossi Y, Hunt S. Adherence to treatment of chronic hepatitis C. *Medicine (Baltimore)*. 2016;95(28):e4151. doi:10.1097/MD.0000000000004151.

[6] Geddawy A, Ibrahim YF, Elbahie NM, Ibrahim MA. Direct acting anti-hepatitis C virus drugs: Clinical pharmacology and future direction. *J Transl Intern Med*. 2017;5(1):8-17. doi:10.1515/jtim-2017-0007.

[7] Missiha SB, Ostrowski M, Heathcote EJ. Disease Progression in Chronic Hepatitis C: Modifiable and Nonmodifiable Factors.

Gastroenterology. 2008;134(6):1699-1714. doi:10.1053/j.gastro. 2008.02.069.
[8] Seeff LB. The history of the "natural history" of hepatitis C (1968-2009). *Liver Int.* 2009;29 Suppl 1:89-99. doi:10.1111/ j.1478-3231.2008.01927.x.
[9] Sarwar S, Khan AA. Sofosbuvir based therapy in Hepatitis C patients with and without cirrhosis: Is there difference? *Pakistan J Med Sci.* 2017;33(1). doi:10.12669/pjms.331.12163.
[10] Thorton K. Evaluation and Prognosis of Patients with Cirrhosis. Hepatatis C Online. https://www.hepatitisc.uw.edu/go/evaluation-staging-monitoring/ evaluation-prognosis-cirrhosis/ core-concept/ all. Published 2018. Accessed March 10, 2019.
[11] Dultz G, Graubard BI, Martin P, et al. Liver transplantation for chronic hepatitis C virus infection in the United States 2002–2014: An analysis of the UNOS/OPTN registry. Gruttadauria S, ed. *PLoS One.* 2017;12(10):e0186898. doi:10.1371/journal.pone.0186898.
[12] Atiemo K, Skaro A, Maddur H, et al. Mortality Risk Factors Among Patients With Cirrhosis and a Low Model for End-Stage Liver Disease Sodium Score (≤15): An Analysis of Liver Transplant Allocation Policy Using Aggregated Electronic Health Record Data. *Am J Transplant.* 2017;17(9):2410-2419. doi:10.1111/ajt.14239.
[13] Kieran JA, Norris S, O'Leary A, et al. Hepatitis C in the era of direct-acting antivirals: Real-world costs of untreated chronic hepatitis C; a cross-sectional study. *BMC Infect Dis.* 2015;15(1). doi:10.1186/ s12879-015-1208-1.
[14] Feld JJ, Jacobson IM, Hézode C, et al. Sofosbuvir and Velpatasvir for HCV Genotype 1, 2, 4, 5, and 6 Infection. *N Engl J Med.* 2015;373(27):2599-2607. doi:10.1056/NEJMoa1512610.
[15] Foster GR, Afdhal N, Roberts SK, et al. Sofosbuvir and Velpatasvir for HCV Genotype 2 and 3 Infection. *N Engl J Med.* 2015;373(27):2608-2617. doi:10.1056/NEJMoa1512612.
[16] Kohli A, Kapoor R, Sims Z, et al. Ledipasvir and sofosbuvir for hepatitis C genotype 4: a proof-of-concept, single-centre, open-label

phase 2a cohort study. *Lancet Infect Dis.* 2015;15(9):1049-1054. doi:10.1016/S1473-3099(15)00157-7.

[17] Afdhal N, Zeuzem S, Kwo P, et al. Ledipasvir and Sofosbuvir for Untreated HCV Genotype 1 Infection. *N Engl J Med.* 2014;370(20):1889-1898. doi:10.1056/NEJMoa1402454.

[18] Powdrill MH, Tchesnokov EP, Kozak RA, et al. Contribution of a mutational bias in hepatitis C virus replication to the genetic barrier in the development of drug resistance. *Proc Natl Acad Sci.* 2011;108(51):20509-20513. doi:10.1073/pnas.1105797108.

[19] Dresch KFN, Mattos AA De, Tovo CV, et al. Impact of the Pegylated-Interferon and Ribavirin Therapy on the Treatment-Related Mortality of Patients with Cirrhosis due to Hepatitis C Virus. *Rev Inst Med Trop Sao Paulo.* 2016;58. doi:10.1590/S1678-9946201658037.

[20] Singh H, Bhatia H, Grewal N, Natt N. Sofosbuvir: A novel treatment option for chronic hepatitis C infection. *J Pharmacol Pharmacother.* 2014;5(4):278. doi:10.4103/0976-500X.142464.

[21] Cuenca-Lopez F, Rivero A, Rivero-Juárez A. Pharmacokinetics and pharmacodynamics of sofosbuvir and ledipasvir for the treatment of hepatitis C. *Expert Opin Drug Metab Toxicol.* 2017;13(1):105-112. doi:10.1080/17425255.2017.1255725.

[22] McGivern DR, Masaki T, Lovell W, Hamlett C, Saalau-Bethell S, Graham B. Protease Inhibitors Block Multiple Functions of the NS3/4A Protease-Helicase during the Hepatitis C Virus Life Cycle. Kirkegaard K, ed. *J Virol.* 2015;89(10):5362-5370. doi:10.1128/JVI.03188-14.

[23] Sesmero E, Thorpe I. Using the Hepatitis C Virus RNA-Dependent RNA Polymerase as a Model to Understand Viral Polymerase Structure, Function and Dynamics. *Viruses.* 2015;7(7):3974-3994. doi:10.3390/v7072808.

[24] Keating GM, Vaidya A. Sofosbuvir: First Global Approval. *Drugs.* 2014;74(2):273-282. doi:10.1007/s40265-014-0179-7.

[25] Jacobson IM, Lawitz E, Gane EJ, et al. Efficacy of 8 Weeks of Sofosbuvir, Velpatasvir, and Voxilaprevir in Patients with Chronic

HCV Infection: 2 Phase 3 Randomized Trials. *Gastroenterology.* 2017;153(1):113-122. doi:10.1053/j.gastro.2017.03.047.

[26] Snyder HS, Ali B, Gonzalez HC, Nair S, Satapathy SK. Efficacy and Safety of Sofosbuvir-Based Direct Acting Antivirals for Hepatitis C in Septuagenarians and Octogenarians. *J Clin Exp Hepatol.* 2017; 7(2):93-96. doi:10.1016/j.jceh.2017.03.009.

[27] Leleu H, Blachier M, Rosa I. Cost-effectiveness of sofosbuvir in the treatment of patients with hepatitis C. *J Viral Hepat.* 2015;22(4):376-383. doi:10.1111/jvh.12311.

[28] Chung RT, Ghany MG, Kim AY, et al. Hepatitis C guidance 2018 update: Aasld-idsa recommendations for testing, managing, and treating Hepatitis C Virus infection. *Clin Infect Dis.* 2018;67(10): 1477-1492. doi:10.1093/cid/ciy585.

[29] Curry MP, O'Leary JG, Bzowej N, et al. Sofosbuvir and Velpatasvir for HCV in Patients with Decompensated Cirrhosis. *N Engl J Med.* 2015;373(27):2618-2628. doi:10.1056/NEJMoa1512614.

[30] Younossi ZM, Stepanova M, Feld J, et al. Sofosbuvir and Velpatasvir Combination Improves Patient-reported Outcomes for Patients With HCV Infection, Without or With Compensated or Decompensated Cirrhosis. *Clin Gastroenterol Hepatol.* 2017;15(3):421-430.e6. doi: 10.1016/j.cgh.2016.10.037.

[31] Messina JP, Humphreys I, Flaxman A, et al. Global distribution and prevalence of hepatitis C virus genotypes. *Hepatology.* 2015;61(1): 77-87. doi:10.1002/hep.27259.

[32] Chahal HS, Marseille EA, Tice JA, et al. Cost-effectiveness of early treatment of hepatitis C virus genotype 1 by stage of liver fibrosis in a US treatment-naive population. *JAMA Intern Med.* 2016;176(1):65-73. doi:10.1001/jamainternmed.2015.6011.

[33] Foster GR, Afdhal N, Roberts SK, et al. Appendix Sofosbuvir and Velpatasvir for HCV Genotype 1, 2, 4, 5, and 6 Infection. *N Engl J Med.* 2015;373(27):2599-2607. doi:10.1056/NEJMoa1512610.

[34] Latt NL, Yanny BT, Gharibian D, Gevorkyan R, Sahota AK. Eight-week ledipasvir/sofosbuvir in non-cirrhotic, treatment-naïve hepatitis C genotype-1 patients with hepatitis C virus-RNA < 6 million: Single

center, real world effectiveness and safety. *World J Gastroenterol.* 2017;23(26):4759. doi:10.3748/wjg.v23.i26.4759.
[35] Gayam V, Tiongson B, Khalid M, et al. Sofosbuvir based regimens in the treatment of chronic hepatitis C genotype 1 infection in African–American patients. *Eur J Gastroenterol Hepatol.* 2018;30 (10):1200-1207. doi:10.1097/MEG.0000000000001233.
[36] Liu CH, Liu CJ, Su TH, et al. Real-world effectiveness and safety of sofosbuvir and ledipasvir with or without ribavirin for patients with hepatitis C virus genotype 1 infection in Taiwan. Kanda T, ed. *PLoS One.* 2018;13(12):e0209299. doi:10.1371/journal.pone.0209299.
[37] Younossi ZM, Stepanova M, Omata M, Mizokami M, Walters M, Hunt S. Quality of life of Japanese patients with chronic hepatitis C treated with ledipasvir and sofosbuvir. *Medicine (Baltimore).* 2016;95(33):e4243. doi:10.1097/MD.0000000000004243.
[38] Kanwal F, Kramer JR, Ilyas J, Duan Z, El-Serag HB. HCV genotype 3 is associated with an increased risk of cirrhosis and hepatocellular cancer in a national sample of U.S. Veterans with HCV. *Hepatology.* 2014;60(1):98-105. doi:10.1002/hep.27095.
[39] Werner CR, Schwarz JM, Egetemeyr DP, et al. Second-generation direct-acting-antiviral hepatitis C virus treatment: Efficacy, safety, and predictors of SVR12. *World J Gastroenterol.* 2016;22(35):8050. doi:10.3748/wjg.v22.i35.8050.
[40] Fathi H, Clark A, Hill NR, Dusheiko G. Effectiveness of current and future regimens for treating genotype 3 hepatitis C virus infection: a large-scale systematic review. *BMC Infect Dis.* 2017;17(1):722. doi: 10.1186/s12879-017-2820-z.
[41] Esteban R, Pineda JA, Calleja JL, et al. Efficacy of Sofosbuvir and Velpatasvir, With and Without Ribavirin, in Patients With Hepatitis C Virus Genotype 3 Infection and Cirrhosis. *Gastroenterology.* 2018;155(4):1120-1127.e4. doi:10.1053/j.gastro.2018.06.042.
[42] Gayam V, Khalid M, Mandal AK, et al. Direct-Acting Antivirals in Chronic Hepatitis C Genotype 4 Infection in Community Care Setting. *Gastroenterol Res.* 2018;11(2):130-137. doi:10.14740/gr999w.

[43] Al Naamani K, Al Sinani S, Descheñes M. Epidemiology and treatment of hepatitis C genotypes 5 and 6. *Can J Gastroenterol.* 2013;27(1).

[44] Bonny C, Roche C, Randl K, et al. 1203 Treatment of interferon-naive patients with HCV genotype 5 with interferon (or PEG-interferon) plus ribavirin results in a very high sustained virological response. *Hepatology.* 2003;38:738-738. doi:10.1016/S0270-9139(03)81241-7.

[45] Legrand-Abravanel F, Sandres-Sauné K, Barange K, et al. Hepatitis C Virus Genotype 5: Epidemiological Characteristics and Sensitivity to Combination Therapy with Interferon-α plus Ribavirin. *J Infect Dis.* 2004;189(8):1397-1400. doi:10.1086/382544.

[46] Bonny C, Fontaine H, Poynard T, et al. Effectiveness of interferon plus ribavirin combination in the treatment of naive patients with hepatitis C virus type 5. A French multicentre retrospective study. *Aliment Pharmacol Ther.* 2006;24(4):593-600. doi:10.1111/j.1365-2036.2006.03018.x.

[47] Antaki N, Hermes A, Hadad M, et al. Efficacy of interferon plus ribavirin in the treatment of hepatitis C virus genotype 5. *J Viral Hepat.* 2008;15(5):383-386. doi:10.1111/j.1365-2893.2007.00946.x.

[48] Dev A. Southeast Asian patients with chronic hepatitis C: The impact of novel genotypes and race on treatment outcome. *Hepatology.* 2002;36(5):1259-1265. doi:10.1053/jhep.2002.36781.

[49] Hui C, Yuen M, Sablon E, Chan AO, Wong BC, Lai C. Interferon and Ribavirin Therapy for Chronic Hepatitis C Virus Genotype 6: A Comparison with Genotype 1. *J Infect Dis.* 2003;187(7):1071-1074. doi:10.1086/368217.

[50] Nguyen MH, Trinh HN, Garcia R, Nguyen G, Lam KD, Keeffe EB. Higher Rate of Sustained Virologic Response in Chronic Hepatitis C Genotype 6 Treated With 48 Weeks Versus 24 Weeks of Peginterferon Plus Ribavirin. *Am J Gastroenterol.* 2008;103(5):1131-1135. doi:10.1111/j.1572-0241.2008.01793.x.

[51] Fung J, Lai C, Hung I, et al. Chronic Hepatitis C Virus Genotype 6 Infection: Response to Pegylated Interferon and Ribavirin. *J Infect Dis*. 2008;198(6):808-812. doi:10.1086/591252.

[52] Lam KD, Trinh HN, Do ST, et al. Randomized controlled trial of pegylated interferon-alfa 2a and ribavirin in treatment-naive chronic hepatitis C genotype 6. *Hepatology*. 2010;52(5):1573-1580. doi:10.1002/hep.23889.

[53] Tangkijvanich P, Komolmit P, Mahachai V, Poovorawan K, Akkarathamrongsin S, Poovorawan Y. Response-guided therapy for patients with hepatitis C virus genotype 6 infection: a pilot study. *J Viral Hepat*. 2012;19(6):423-430. doi:10.1111/j.1365-2893.2011.01566.x.

[54] Thu Thuy PT, Bunchorntavakul C, Tan Dat H, Rajender Reddy K. A randomized trial of 48 versus 24 weeks of combination pegylated interferon and ribavirin therapy in genotype 6 chronic hepatitis C. *J Hepatol*. 2012;56(5):1012-1018. doi:10.1016/j.jhep.2011.12.020.

[55] Abergel A, Asselah T, Metivier S, et al. Ledipasvir-sofosbuvir in patients with hepatitis C virus genotype 5 infection: an open-label, multicentre, single-arm, phase 2 study. *Lancet Infect Dis*. 2016;16(4):459-464. doi:10.1016/S1473-3099(15)00529-0.

[56] Wong RJ, Nguyen MT, Trinh HN, et al. Community-based real-world treatment outcomes of sofosbuvir/ledipasvir in Asians with chronic hepatitis C virus genotype 6 in the United States. *J Viral Hepat*. 2017;24(1):17-21. doi:10.1111/jvh.12609.

[57] Centers for Disease Control and Prevention. Estimated HIV Incidence and Prevalence in the United States (2010–2016). https://www.cdc.gov/ hiv/ library/ slidesets/ index.html. Published 2019. Accessed March 10, 2019.

[58] Hall HI. Estimation of HIV Incidence in the United States. *JAMA*. 2008;300(5):520. doi:10.1001/jama.300.5.520.

[59] Chen JY, Feeney ER, Chung RT. HCV and HIV co-infection: mechanisms and management. *Nat Rev Gastroenterol Hepatol*. 2014;11(6):362-371. doi:10.1038/nrgastro.2014.17.

[60] Kim DY. Efficacy of Direct-Acting Antivirals in Patients with Hepatitis C Virus/Human Immunodeficiency Virus Coinfection: A Gap between Clinical Trial and Real Practice. *Gut Liver*. 2018; 12(6):609-610. doi:10.5009/gnl18418.

[61] Gayam V, Hossain MR, Khalid M, et al. Real-World Clinical Efficacy and Tolerability of Direct-Acting Antivirals in Hepatitis C Monoinfection Compared to Hepatitis C/Human Immunodeficiency Virus Coinfection in a Community Care Setting. *Gut Liver*. 2018; 12(6):694-703. doi:10.5009/gnl18004.

[62] Wyles DL, Ruane PJ, Sulkowski MS, et al. Daclatasvir plus Sofosbuvir for HCV in Patients Coinfected with HIV-1. *N Engl J Med*. 2015;373(8):714-725. doi:10.1056/NEJMoa1503153

[63] Zipprich A, Garcia-tsao G, Rogowski S, Fleig WE, Seufferlein T, Dollinger MM. Prognostic indicators of survival in patients with compensated and decompensated cirrhosis. *Liver Int*. 2012;32(9): 1407-14.

In: The Pharmacological Guide to Sofosbuvir   ISBN: 978-1-53616-476-3
Editor: Vijay Gayam   © 2019 Nova Science Publishers, Inc.

Chapter 4

MANAGEMENT OF HCV INFECTION WITH SOFOSBUVIR-BASED REGIMENS IN PATIENTS WITH MEDICAL CO-MORBIDITIES

Amrendra Kumar Mandal[1,*], *MD,*
Venu Madhav Konala[2], *MD, Sreedhar Adapa*[3], *MD,*
Srikanth Naramala[4], *MD, Benjamin Tiongson*[1], *MD*
and Vijay Gayam[1], *MD*

[1]Department of Internal Medicine, Interfaith Medical Center, Brooklyn, NY, US
[2]Department of Internal Medicine, Division of Medical Oncology, Ashland Bellefonte Cancer Center, Ashland, KY, US
[3]Division of Nephrology, The Nephrology group, Fresno, CA, US
[4]Department of Internal Medicine, Division of Rheumatology Adventist Medical Center, Hanford, CA, US

---

* Corresponding Author's E-mail: Amandal@interfaithmedical.com

ABSTRACT

Hepatitis C virus infection is one of the common causes of chronic liver disease, with approximately 71 million infected individuals across the world. The availability of newer direct-acting antiviral regimens now provides physicians worldwide with the opportunity to simplify, and thereby facilitate, treatment access at a reasonable cost. Hepatitis C virus can progress to cirrhosis, decompensation, and eventually hepatorenal syndrome and hepatocellular carcinoma. Liver transplantation is the treatment of choice for patients with end-stage liver disease, although it can recur because of graft infection post-transplantation in the absence of prevention; the life of the graft and survival are reduced in patients with recurrent hepatitis C. The treatment of chronic hepatitis C in a patient with medical co-morbidities brings certain challenges. One should take into account changes in drug metabolism in patients with renal impairment or decompensated liver cirrhosis; also drug-drug interactions in transplanted patients should be considered. Sofosbuvir is a backbone for the treatment of chronic hepatitis C virus infection. However, it should be used with caution in a patient with a glomerular filtration rate of <30 mL/min. Patients with low baseline renal function have a higher frequency of anemia, worsening renal dysfunction, and more severe adverse events, but treatment responses remain high and comparable to those without renal impairment. Direct-acting antivirals are recommended for patients with MELD score <20 or MELD exception points (when the expected waiting time is less than one year). In this chapter, we elaborate on the role of direct-acting antivirals in patients with chronic hepatitis c virus infections with co-morbid medical conditions, and the strategies to approach in these settings.

Keywords: hepatitis C virus, sofosbuvir, sustained virologic response, cirrhosis, liver transplantation

ABBREVIATIONS

DAA	Direct-Acting Antivirals
CTP	Child-Turcotte-Pugh
MELD	Model for End-Stage Liver Disease
HCC	Hepatocellular Carcinoma
VEL	Velpatasvir

SOF   Sofosbuvir
CKD   Chronic Kidney Disease
HCV   Hepatitis C Virus
ESRD   End-Stage Renal Disease
MTCT   Mother-to-Child-Transmission
HIV   Human Immunodeficiency Syndrome
SVR   Sustained Virologic Response
LT   Liver Transplantation
eGFR   estimated Glomerular Filtration Rate
HBV   Hepatitis B Virus
AASLD   American Association for the Study of Liver Disease
IDSA   Infectious Disease Society of America
LDV   Ledipasvir
RBV   Ribavirin
DCV   Daclatasvir
FDA   Food and Drug Association

1. INTRODUCTION

In persons with decompensated cirrhosis, most patients receiving direct-acting antiviral (DAA) therapy experience improvement in clinical and biochemical indicators of liver disease between baseline and post-treatment week 12, including patients with Child-Turcotte-Pugh (CTP) class C cirrhosis [1]. The predictors of improvement or decline have not been identified, though patients with a Model for End-Stage Liver Disease (MELD) score >20 or severe portal hypertension complications may be less likely to improve and might be better served by transplantation than treatment [2].

Real-world data comparing DAA response rates demonstrate that patients with cirrhosis and hepatocellular carcinoma (HCC) have lower sustained virologic response (SVR) rates than cirrhotic patients without HCC [3]. In a large Veteran's Affair study including sofosbuvir (SOF) based and other DAA based regimens, overall SVR rates were 91% in patients without HCC vs. 74% in those with HCC [4].

To date, there have been no studies evaluating the safety and efficacy of the fixed-dose combination of sofosbuvir (400 mg)/velpatasvir (VEL) (100 mg) in liver transplant (LT) recipients. For this reason, very limited recommendations on its use post-LT can be made. However, with no treatment options for LT recipients with genotype 2 or 3 infections who have decompensated cirrhosis, expert opinion led to the recommendation to use SOF/VEL with weight-based ribavirin for these patients [5]. Similarly, recognition of the need for alternative options for patients with genotype 2 or 3 infections and cirrhosis—especially those who are treatment-experienced—led to the inclusion of SOF/VEL as an alternative regimen for patients with compensated cirrhosis [5]. The safety of SOF and other NS5A inhibitors has been demonstrated.

Chronic hepatitis C is also independently associated with the development of chronic kidney disease (CKD) [6]. A meta-analysis published in 2015 demonstrated that chronic Hepatitis C Virus (HCV) infection was associated with a 51% increase in the risk of proteinuria and a 43% increase in the incidence of CKD [7]. There is also a higher risk of progression to end-stage renal disease (ESRD) in persons with chronic HCV infection and CKD, and an increased risk of all-cause mortality in persons on dialysis. Several additional reports have described successful outcomes with combination direct-acting antiviral (DAA) therapy in kidney transplant recipients [8].

During pregnancy, Hepatitis C Mother-to-child transmission (MTCT) occurs at an overall rate of 5% to 15%, with the number that progress to the chronic infection being 3% to 5% [9, 10]. No specific risk factor predicts transmission and no specific intervention (e.g., antiviral, mode of delivery, or others) has been demonstrated to reduce transmission—except for suppression of HIV replication in women with Human Immunodeficiency Virus (HIV)/HCV co-infection [11]. Given the potential associated risk of MTCT, it is advisable to avoid invasive procedures (e.g., fetal scalp monitors and forceps delivery). However, treatment during pregnancy is not recommended due to the lack of safety and efficacy data. For women of reproductive age with known HCV infection, antiviral therapy is recommended before considering pregnancy - whenever practical and feasible, to reduce the risk of HCV transmission to future offspring [5]. In a retrospective real-world study in patients with HCV infections treated with SOF-based regimens, the SVR12 of patients with medical conditions such as people living with acquired Immunodeficiency syndrome with the presence of comorbidities (e.g., hypertension, diabetes, compensated cirrhosis or previous treatment) was not affected [12]. In another real-world study evaluating the safety and efficacy of patients in SOF-based regimens, it was demonstrated that there was an associated statistical difference in SVR 12 rates in patients with low platelet count and HIV/HCV co-infection [13, 14].

2. SOFOSBUVIR-BASED REGIMENS IN THE TREATMENT OF DECOMPENSATED LIVER CIRRHOSIS

Patients with decompensated cirrhosis and indications for LT with a MELD score of ≥18–20 will benefit from transplantation first and antiviral treatment after transplantation. This is due to the probability of significant improvement in liver function, and being removed from the LT list is low [15]. However, if the waiting list for LT is more than 6 months, then treatment should be offered to patients in the appropriate treatment facility center. Three different regimens are discussed below. The recommended treatment regimens for genotypes 1,4,5 or 6 are highlighted in Table 1, and for Table 2 for genotype 2 and 3.

Table 1. The recommended treatment regimen for patients with HCV infection Genotype 1,4,5 or 6 and with Decompensated Cirrhosis

Regimen	Comments
Daily fixed dose of ledipasvir (90 mg)/sofosbuvir (400 mg) with a low initial dose of ribavirin (600 mg)	Increase ribavirin as tolerated.
A daily fixed dose of sofosbuvir (400 mg)/velpatasvir (100 mg) with weight-based ribavirin	The low initial dose of ribavirin (600mg) is recommended for patients with CTP class C cirrhosis; increase as tolerated.
Daily daclatasvir (60 mg) plus sofosbuvir (400 mg) with a low initial dose of ribavirin (600 mg)	Increase ribavirin as tolerated* For genotype 1 or 4 only for ribavirin ineligible patients.

Note: Typical duration of treatment is 12 weeks; 24 weeks duration of therapy is recommended for patients who are ineligible to receive ribavirin, had prior treatment failure with sofosbuvir or NS5A-based treatment failure.

* 24 weeks for prior sofosbuvir-based treatment failure only.

Source: American Association for the study of liver diseases- Infectious Disease Society of America (AASLD-IDSA) HCV Guidance Panel [16].

Table 2. Recommended treatment regimen for patients with HCV infection Genotype 2 or 3 and with decompensated cirrhosis

Regimen	Comments
Daily fixed dose of sofosbuvir (400 mg)/velpatasvir (100 mg) with weight-based ribavirin	Increase ribavirin as tolerated.
Daily daclatasvir (60 mg) plus sofosbuvir (400 mg) with a low initial dose of ribavirin (600 mg)	Increase ribavirin as tolerated *

Note: Typical duration of treatment is 12 weeks; 24 weeks duration of therapy is recommended for patients who are: ineligible to receive ribavirin, with prior use of sofosbuvir or failure of NS5A-based treatment regimens

* Not approved by the Food and Drug Association for Genotype 2 infection.

Source: AASLD-IDSA HCV Guidance Panel [16].

2.1. HCV Treatment for Genotypes 1, 4, 5 or 6 with Decompensated Cirrhosis

2.1.1. Ledipasvir/Sofosbuvir

In phase 2 SOLAR-1 clinical trial, investigators studied the combination of ledipasvir (LDV) (90 mg)/SOF (400 mg) plus ribavirin

(RBV) (initial dose of 600 mg) in patients with genotype 1 or 4 [17]. SVR rates were 86% and 87%, for 12 weeks and 24 weeks of antiviral therapy respectively, in CTP class C patients. After completion of therapy, relapse occurred in 8% and 5% of the 12- and 24-week groups, respectively. In the majority of the patients with CTP class B or C cirrhosis, the MELD and CTP scores decreased between baseline and post-treatment at week-4 [17].

In the multi-center SOLAR-2 trial, patients with decompensated cirrhosis (CTP class B or C) showed SVR 12 of 90%. However, SVR 24 showed further improvement with 98% in CTP class B but was lower in 77% CTP class C [1].

Both SOLAR-1 AND SOLAR-2 clinical trials have shown minor adverse events, which were most likely attributed to ribavirin. However, serious adverse events occurred in approximately 28% of patients with decompensated cirrhosis [1, 17]. Therapy was discontinued in about 7-8%, and relapse after completion of therapy was seen in only 6% in 12 weeks of therapy as compared to < 2% in 24-week regimens. Results from the previous two trials were also supported by the multicenter trial conducted in France using the regimen of LDV/SOF plus RBV [18].

2.1.2. Sofosbuvir/Velpatasvir

In phase 3 ASTRAL-4 trial, HCV infected patients of any genotype with decompensated cirrhosis classified as CTP class B were recruited and divided to the three groups: SOF 400 mg/VEL 100mg for 12 weeks, SOF/VEL plus RBV for 12 weeks, and SOF/VEL for 24 weeks respectively. The highest efficacy was achieved with the SOF/VEL + RBV regimen, with 94% SVR rate, then followed by the SOF/VEL for 24 weeks with 86% and lastly, the SOF/VEL group with 83% [19]. At post-treatment week 12, 47% (n=117/250) of patients had an improvement in CTP score, 42% (n=106/250) had no change, and 11% (n=27/250) had an increased CTP score. Three percent (n=9/250) died due to several causes; however, no death was attributed to DAA. Serious adverse events were reported in 16% to 19% of the treated patients [19].

2.1.3. Daclatasvir + Sofosbuvir

In the phase 3 ALLY-1 trial, researchers evaluated the efficacy and safety of 12 weeks of daclatasvir (DCV) (60 mg) and SOF (400 mg) along with RBV (600 mg - 1000 mg as tolerated) among patients with cirrhosis (CTP class A, B, or C) or HCV recurrence after LT. SVR12 rates were achieved in 92% with CTP class A cirrhosis, 94% with class B, and 56% with class C cirrhosis [20].

In a real-world study by Foster, 91% of the patients received RBV; only 6% discontinued RBV, but 20% required an RBV dose reduction. MELD scores improved in 42% of treated patients and worsened in 11% [21]. There were 14 deaths, and 26% developed serious adverse event (none related to DAA). These data highlight the lower efficacy and increased safety concerns when treating patients with more advanced liver failure.

2.2. HCV Treatment for Genotypes 2 or 3 with Decompensated Cirrhosis

HCV treatment, as recommended by the AASLD-IDSA, is highlighted in Table 2.

2.2.1. Sofosbuvir/Velpatasvir

ASTRAL-4 evaluated CTP class B cirrhosis for genotype 2 HCV infections and found that SVR 12 rate was 100% for all study groups (SOF/VEL 12, n=4/4, SOF/VEL + RBV n=5/5, SOF/VEL 24, n=4/4) while CTP class B cirrhosis with genotype 3 infection had an SVR rate of 85% (n=11/13) for 12 weeks of SOF/VEL plus RBV. HCV genotype 3-infected patients especially benefitted from ribavirin with the regimen [22].

In the case of ribavirin ineligibility, SOF/VEL for 24 weeks is currently recommended. However, SOF/VEL has not been studied in CTP class C patients [16].

2.2.2. Daclatasvir + Sofosbuvir

DCV and SOF for 12 weeks were approved by the FDA for the treatment of HCV genotype 3 infections in patients with and without cirrhosis, although it was not approved for the treatment of genotype 2 infections. However, the ALLY-1 study supported DCV/SOF and RBV in patients with genotype 2 or 3 infection who have decompensated cirrhosis [23]. Eighty percent of patients with decompensated cirrhosis (CTP class B/C) were treated with DCV/SOF plus RBV, and SVR rates were 80% for genotype 2 patients and 83% for genotype 3 patients with advanced cirrhosis [23].

The trial from the Spanish study for DCV/SOF with or without RBV in genotype 3-infected patients (the majority of patients receiving 24 weeks), showed SVR12 of 94% in both CTP class A and CTP class B/C patients [24].

However, compared to CTP class A patients, the CTP class B/C patients had more frequent serious adverse events (16.7% vs. 3.6%) and had episodes of hepatic decompensation (5.2% vs. 2.3%).

Currently, DAA is invariably used for HCV infections, however in the past with interferon-based regimens; it was not used in the patients with decompensated cirrhosis (moderate or severe hepatic impairment, CTP class B or C) because of the potential for worsening hepatic decompensation [25].

Limited data exist for the use of simeprevir in patients with CTP class B cirrhosis [26, 27].

3. SOFOSBUVIR-BASED REGIMENS IN THE TREATMENT OF RECURRENT HCV INFECTION POST-LIVER TRANSPLANTATION

Treatment of HCV infection pre-transplant in patients awaiting LT should be treated with two major goals: prevention of liver graft infection after transplantation by achieving SVR 12/24 and improvement in the liver function before LT. Recommended treatment regimens for post-LT for genotype 1,4,5, or 6 is presented in Table 3 and Table 4 for genotype 2 and 3.

Table 3. Post liver transplantation: Genotype 1, 4, 5, or 6 infection

Regimen	Comments
Fixed-dose combination of ledipasvir (90 mg)/sofosbuvir (400 mg) with weight-based ribavirin	With or without compensated cirrhosis Start with a low initial dose of ribavirin (600mg, increase as tolerated) for patients with decompensated cirrhosis.
Daclatasvir (60 mg) plus sofosbuvir (400 mg) with a low initial dose of ribavirin (600 mg, increase as tolerated)	Alternative treatment option
Simeprevir (150 mg) plus sofosbuvir (400 mg) with or without weight-based ribavirin	Alternative treatment option for HCV genotype 1 or 4 infections only

Note: Treatment duration is daily for 12 weeks.
Source: AASLD-IDSA HCV Guidance Panel [16].

Table 4. Post-liver transplantation: Genotype 2 or 3 infection with or without cirrhosis

Regimen	Comments
daclatasvir (60 mg) plus sofosbuvir (400 mg) with ribavirin	Start with a low initial dose of ribavirin (600mg, increase as tolerated)
a fixed-dose combination of sofosbuvir (400 mg)/velpatasvir (100 mg) with weight-based ribavirin	Alternative treatment option

Note: Treatment duration is daily for 12 weeks.
Source: AASLD-IDSA HCV Guidance Panel [16].

3.1. Ledipasvir/Sofosbuvir

The Trial from SOLAR-1 has shown SVR rates of 96% and 98% in LT patients without cirrhosis in the 12- and 24-week treatment arms, respectively. In patients with compensated cirrhosis, SVR was achieved in 96%. However, efficacy was lower in patients with CTP class B or C cirrhosis post LT [17].

SVR rates were 86% and 88% in the 12- and 24-week treatment arms, respectively in CTP class B cirrhosis and 60% and 75% in the 12- and 24-week treatment arms, respectively in CTP class C patients. Ten percent mortality rate was seen among patients with CTP class B or class C cirrhosis [17].

Similar results were achieved using an identical study design in the SOLAR-2 study, conducted in Europe, Australia, Canada, and New Zealand [28].

Most clinical trials to date have emphasized on patients having DAA at least 6 months post-LT [29]. SVR12 post-LT was attained in 88% [15, 16] of patients [29]. Earlier treatment for HCV may be started if the patient is on stable immunosuppression and has recovered from postoperative complications.

In general, these real-world data indicate high SVR rates in the absence of RBV in LT patients. However, we should bear in mind that RBV is recommended for patients with unfavorable baseline characteristics such as cirrhosis, prior treatment experience, and RBV-free therapy is recommended for patients with a favorable baseline profile.

3.2. Daclatasvir /Sofosbuvir

The phase 3 open-label ALLY-1 trial evaluated the efficacy and safety of a subgroup of patients with HCV recurrence after LT. SVR 12 rates was 94% and 83% in genotype 1 and 3, respectively [23]. Overall, DCV-containing regimens appear to be well tolerated.

3.3. Sofosbuvir/Velpatasvir

SOF/VEL-based regimens have not been evaluated in terms of safety and efficacy in LT recipients. Hence, few recommendations on its use post-LT can be derived.

However, with no treatment options for LT recipients with HCV genotype 2 or 3 infections who have decompensated cirrhosis, expert opinion led to the recommendation to use SOF/VEL with weight-based RBV for these patients [16].

4. HCV TREATMENT IN PATIENTS WITH RENAL IMPAIRMENT

It has been found that the development of CKD is independently associated with Chronic Hepatitis C infection [6, 30]. In a meta-analysis analyzing risks of HCV and CKD, it was seen that there was a 51% risk of proteinuria and 43% risk of CKD due to chronic HCV. Furthermore, it was also elucidated in the study that there was a greater risk of development of ESRD for persons with HCV infection as compared to those without HCV or Hepatitis B infection (HBV), and an increased risk of all-cause mortality for persons on dialysis [7]. AASLD treatment recommendations for HCV treatment in CKD are highlighted in Table 5.

Table 5. Recommendations for patients with Chronic Kidney Disease stage 1, 2 and 3

Regimens	Comments
Fixed-dose combination of ledipasvir (90 mg)/ sofosbuvir (400 mg)	daily for 12 weeks.
Fixed-dose combination of sofosbuvir (400 mg)/ velpatasvir (100 mg)	daily for 12 weeks.
Fixed-dose combination of sofosbuvir (400 mg)/ velpatasvir (100 mg)/voxilaprevir (100 mg)	daily for 12 weeks.

Note: No sofosbuvir-based regimen recommendation for CKD stages 4 and 5.
Source: AASLD-IDSA HCV Guidance Panel [16].

There was no substantial evidence that supports an appropriate cut-off dose for sofosbuvir in patients with an estimated glomerular filtration rate (eGFR) <30 mL/min. However, recently, there is increasing evidence on the use of SOF-based regimens for this population [31, 32].

The HCV-TARGET study (prospective, observational cohort study) evaluated the use of DAA for patients from North America and Europe. Overall, the regimens were well tolerated with no increased concern for discontinuation due to low eGFRs [33]. There were higher SVR12 rates among the eGFR groups but at the expense of progressive worsening in the renal function with an eGFR <30 mL/min, which suggests that those groups of patients require close monitoring [33].

5. SOFOSBUVIR BASED THERAPY IN PATIENTS UNDERGOING RENAL TRANSPLANT

An open-label clinical trial by Colombo *et al.* evaluated recently the combination of LDV (90 mg)/SOF (400 mg) in renal transplant recipients who had completed 6 months post-renal-transplant [34]. The majority of patients were HCV genotype 1 and 4 infections. Among them, 69% were treatment-naive, and 15% had compensated cirrhosis with an overall SVR12 of 100% (n=114/114). Common adverse events noted were headache (n=22, 19%), asthenia (n=16, 14%), and fatigue (n=11, 10%); while serious adverse events occurred in 13 patients (11%). One patient discontinued treatment due to syncope.

Recommended SOF-based treatment regimens for renal transplant patients are shown in Table 6.

Table 6. Sofosbuvir-based regimens for renal transplant patients

Regimens	Comments
ledipasvir (90 mg)/sofosbuvir (400 mg)	with or without compensated cirrhosis for HCV Genotypes 1 and 4
daclatasvir (60 mg) plus sofosbuvir (400 mg) plus a low initial dose of ribavirin (600 mg, increase as tolerated)	Alternative treatment For HCV Genotypes 2, 3, 5, and 6

Note: Treatment duration is daily for 12 weeks.
Source: AASLD-IDSA HCV Guidance Panel [16].

6. SOFOSBUVIR-BASED REGIMENS FOR THE SIMULTANEOUS TREATMENT OF LIVER AND KIDNEY TRANSPLANT PATIENTS

The real-world HCV-TARGET study evaluated the efficacy of DAA therapy in patients with kidney transplant as well as for dual liver-kidney transplant [35]. The investigators included several regimens, including SOF/LDV ± RBV; SOF plus DCV ± RBV, which demonstrated an SVR12 rate of 90.9% in dual liver and kidney transplant recipients. Based on this study, SOF-based regimens are recommended and have exhibited excellent efficacy and safety.

7. SOFOSBUVIR-BASED REGIMENS IN PATIENTS WITH HEPATOCELLULAR CARCINOMA

There is controversy in the exact timing to start DAA in patients with HCC. The argument is either before or after LT in HCC patients without cirrhosis but who is a candidate for LT [36].

Table 7. Sofosbuvir-based Regimens and its Interactions with Calcineurin Inhibitors

Regimens	Cyclosporine	Tacrolimus
Sofosbuvir	4.5-fold ↑ in SOF AUC, but GS-331007 metabolite unchanged; no a priori dose adjustment	No interaction observed; no a priori dose adjustment
Sofosbuvir/velpatasvir/voxilaprevir	9.4-fold ↑ in VOX AUC; the combination is not recommended	No data; no a priori dose adjustment

AUC = Area under the curve
Source: AASLD-IDSA HCV Guidance Panel [16].

Lower SVR rates have been observed in patients with HCC treated with SOF-based regimens with or without RBV, than in patients without HCC or in patients with HCC treated after LT (74% vs. 91% and 94%, respectively) [4].

Post-LT treatment of HCV was reported to be cost-effective in patients with HCC [37]. In this population, pre- or post-LT antiviral treatment indications are like those in patients who do not have HCC, previous history of DAA treatment and compensated or decompensated cirrhosis [37].

8. Drug Interactions of Sofosbuvir-Based Regimens with Transplant Medications

DCV area under the curve is 40% and 5%, respectively; despite cyclosporine and tacrolimus increases, these changes are not clinically significant [5]. DCV cause minor changes in calcineurin inhibitor, mammalian target of rapamycin (mTOR) inhibitor, steroid, or mycophenolate levels [5].

VEL is a substrate for CYP3A4, CYP2C8, and CYP2B6 and is moderately affected by potent inhibitors and, to a greater extent, potent inducers of enzyme/drug transporter systems [38]. Based on this profile, clinically significant drug-drug interactions would not be expected for co-administration of SOF/VEL or LDV with common immunosuppressive agents (e.g., tacrolimus, cyclosporine, corticosteroids, mycophenolate mofetil, or everolimus).

9. HCV Treatment in Pregnancy

Up to 29,000 HCV-infected women were estimated to have delivered every year between 2011 and 2014 [39]. Recently, there is an increasing trend in HCV infections among young adults, including women of childbearing age [40]. HCV-infected women of reproductive age should be initiated by DAA-based regimens before planning for pregnancy, which could improve the health of the mother and reduce the risk of MTCT [5].

The safety of DAAs in pregnancy is not well understood, and there is no evidence on the effect of DAAs on male or female fertility [41]. However, RBV is contraindicated in pregnancy due to its known teratogenicity [42]. Moreover, the risk for teratogenicity continues for up to 6 months even after stopping RBV – and it also applies to women taking RBV and female partners of men taking RBV [42].

Conclusion

SOF-based regimens have emerged as an effective combination therapy for HCV infections. Despite these innovations, co-morbid medical conditions continue to complicate treatment and make it a challenge for healthcare professionals. One should be aware of patients with hepatic decompensation, HCC, and renal impairments in treating chronic HCV infection, as well as monitoring graft survival due to a chance of decline caused by recurrent HCV infection post-LT. Lastly, although since limited data can be found on drug-drug interactions between SOF-based treatments and LT medications, use of these medications in conjunction with one another should be approached with caution. Further research can be done to influence the future management of these situations.

References

[1] Manns M, Samuel D, Gane EJ, Mutimer D, McCaughan G, Buti M, et al. Ledipasvir and sofosbuvir plus ribavirin in patients with genotype 1 or 4 hepatitis C virus infection and advanced liver disease: a multicentre, open-label, randomized, phase 2 trial. *The Lancet Infectious Diseases.* 2016;16(6):685-97.

[2] Terrault NA, McCaughan GW, Curry MP, Gane E, Fagiuoli S, Fung JY, et al. International liver transplantation society consensus statement on hepatitis C management in liver transplant candidates. *Transplantation*. 2017;101(5):945-55.

[3] Prenner SB, VanWagner LB, Flamm SL, Salem R, Lewandowski RJ, Kulik L. Hepatocellular carcinoma decreases the chance of successful hepatitis C virus therapy with direct-acting antivirals. *Journal of hepatology*. 2017;66(6):1173-81.

[4] Beste LA, Green PK, Berry K, Kogut MJ, Allison SK, Ioannou GN. Effectiveness of hepatitis C antiviral treatment in a USA cohort of veteran patients with hepatocellular carcinoma. *Journal of hepatology*. 2017;67(1):32-9.

[5] Hepatitis C Guidance 2018 Update: AASLD-IDSA Recommendations for Testing, Managing, and Treating Hepatitis C Virus Infection. *Clinical infectious diseases: an official publication of the Infectious Diseases Society of America*. 2018;67(10):1477-92.

[6] Rogal SS, Yan P, Rimland D, Re VL, Al-Rowais H, Fried L, et al. Incidence and progression of chronic kidney disease after hepatitis C seroconversion: results from ERCHIVES. *Digestive diseases and sciences*. 2016;61(3):930-6.

[7] Lee JJ, Lin MY, Chang JS, Hung CC, Chang JM, Chen HC, et al. Hepatitis C virus infection increases risk of developing end-stage renal disease using competing risk analysis. *PloS one*. 2014;9(6): e100790.

[8] Sawinski D, Kaur N, Ajeti A, Trofe-Clark J, Lim M, Bleicher M, et al. Successful treatment of hepatitis C in renal transplant recipients with direct-acting antiviral agents. *American Journal of Transplantation*. 2016;16(5):1588-95.

[9] Jhaveri R, Hashem M, El-Kamary SS, Saleh DaA, Sharaf SA, El-Mougy F, et al., editors. Hepatitis C virus (HCV) vertical transmission in 12-month-old infants born to HCV-infected women and assessment of maternal risk factors. *Open forum infectious diseases;* 2015: Oxford University Press.

[10] Shebl FM, El-Kamary SS, Saleh DaA, Abdel-Hamid M, Mikhail N, Allam A, et al. Prospective cohort study of mother-to-infant infection and clearance of hepatitis C in rural Egyptian villages. *Journal of medical virology.* 2009;81(6):1024-31.
[11] Checa Cabot CA, Stoszek SK, Quarleri J, Losso MH, Ivalo S, Peixoto MF, et al. Mother-to-child transmission of hepatitis C virus (HCV) among HIV/HCV-coinfected women. Journal of the pediatric infectious diseases society. 2012;2(2):126-35.
[12] Gayam V, Tiongson B, Khalid M, Mandal AK, Mukhtar O, Gill A, et al. Sofosbuvir based regimens in the treatment of chronic hepatitis C genotype 1 infection in African–American patients: a community-based retrospective cohort study. *European journal of gastroenterology & hepatology.* 2018;30(10):1200.
[13] Gayam V, Mandal AK, Khalid M, Mukhtar O, Gill A, Garlapati P, et al. Sofosbuvir Based Regimens in the Treatment of Chronic Hepatitis C with Compensated Liver Cirrhosis in Community Care Setting. *International journal of hepatology.* 2018;2018.
[14] Gayam V, Hossain MR, Khalid M, Chakaraborty S, Mukhtar O, Dahal S, et al. Real-world clinical efficacy and tolerability of direct-acting antivirals in hepatitis C monoinfection compared to hepatitis C/human immunodeficiency virus coinfection in a community care setting. *Gut and liver.* 2018;12(6):694.
[15] EASL Recommendations on Treatment of Hepatitis C 2018. *Journal of hepatology.* 2018;69(2):461-511.
[16] Panel A-IHG. Hepatitis C Guidance 2018 Update: AASLD-IDSA Recommendations for Testing, Managing, and Treating Hepatitis C Virus Infection. *Clin Infect Dis.* 2018;67(10):1477-92.
[17] Charlton M, Everson GT, Flamm SL, Kumar P, Landis C, Brown Jr RS, et al. Ledipasvir and sofosbuvir plus ribavirin for treatment of HCV infection in patients with advanced liver disease. *Gastroenterology.* 2015;149(3):649-59.
[18] Yoshida EM, Kwo P, Agarwal K, Duvoux C, Durand F, Peck-Radosavljevic M, et al. Persistence of virologic response after liver transplant in hepatitis C patients treated with ledipasvir/sofosbuvir

plus ribavirin pretransplant. *Annals of hepatology.* 2017;16(3):375-81.

[19] Curry MP, O'Leary JG, Bzowej N, Muir AJ, Korenblat KM, Fenkel JM, et al. Sofosbuvir and Velpatasvir for HCV in Patients with Decompensated Cirrhosis. *N Engl J Med.* 2015;373(27):2618-28.

[20] Poordad F, Hezode C, Trinh R, Kowdley KV, Zeuzem S, Agarwal K, et al. ABT-450/r–ombitasvir and dasabuvir with ribavirin for hepatitis C with cirrhosis. *New England Journal of Medicine.* 2014;370(21):1973-82.

[21] Foster GR, Afdhal N, Roberts SK, Bräu N, Gane EJ, Pianko S, et al. Sofosbuvir and velpatasvir for HCV genotype 2 and 3 infection. *New England Journal of Medicine.* 2015;373(27):2608-17.

[22] Curry MP, O'Leary JG, Bzowej N, Muir AJ, Korenblat KM, Fenkel JM, et al. Sofosbuvir and velpatasvir for HCV in patients with decompensated cirrhosis. *New England Journal of Medicine.* 2015; 373(27):2618-28.

[23] Poordad F, Schiff ER, Vierling JM, Landis C, Fontana RJ, Yang R, et al. Daclatasvir with sofosbuvir and ribavirin for hepatitis C virus infection with advanced cirrhosis or post-liver transplantation recurrence. *Hepatology.* 2016;63(5):1493-505.

[24] Alonso S, Riveiro-Barciela M, Fernandez I, Rincón D, Real Y, Llerena S, et al. Effectiveness and safety of sofosbuvir-based regimens plus an NS 5A inhibitor for patients with HCV genotype 3 infection and cirrhosis. Results of a multicenter real-life cohort. *Journal of viral hepatitis.* 2017;24(4):304-11.

[25] Modi AA, Nazario H, Trotter JF, Gautam M, Weinstein J, Mantry P, et al. Safety and efficacy of simeprevir plus sofosbuvir with or without ribavirin in patients with decompensated genotype 1 hepatitis C cirrhosis. *Liver transplantation : official publication of the American Association for the Study of Liver Diseases and the International Liver Transplantation Society.* 2016;22(3):281-6.

[26] Modi AA, Nazario H, Trotter JF, Gautam M, Weinstein J, Mantry P, et al. Safety and efficacy of simeprevir plus sofosbuvir with or

without ribavirin in patients with decompensated genotype 1 hepatitis C cirrhosis. *Liver transplantation.* 2016;22(3):281-6.
[27] Lawitz E, Mangia A, Wyles D, Rodriguez-Torres M, Hassanein T, Gordon SC, et al. Sofosbuvir for previously untreated chronic hepatitis C infection. *New England Journal of Medicine.* 2013;368 (20):1878-87.
[28] Yoshida EM, Kwo P, Agarwal K, Duvoux C, Durand F, Peck-Radosavljevic M, et al. Persistence of Virologic Response after Liver Transplant in Hepatitis C Patients Treated with Ledipasvir / Sofosbuvir Plus Ribavirin Pretransplant. *Annals of hepatology.* 2017;16(3):375-81.
[29] Levitsky J, Verna EC, O'Leary JG, Bzowej NH, Moonka DK, Hyland RH, et al. Perioperative ledipasvir–sofosbuvir for HCV in liver-transplant recipients. *New England Journal of Medicine.* 2016;375(21):2106-8.
[30] Fabrizi F, Verdesca S, Messa P, Martin P. Hepatitis C virus infection increases the risk of developing chronic kidney disease: a systematic review and meta-analysis. *Digestive diseases and sciences.* 2015;60(12):3801-13.
[31] Desnoyer A, Pospai D, Lê MP, Gervais A, Heurgué-Berlot A, Laradi A, et al. Pharmacokinetics, safety and efficacy of a full dose sofosbuvir-based regimen given daily in hemodialysis patients with chronic hepatitis C. *Journal of hepatology.* 2016;65(1):40-7.
[32] Nazario HE, Ndungu M, Modi AA. Sofosbuvir and simeprevir in hepatitis C genotype 1-patients with end-stage renal disease on haemodialysis or GFR< 30 ml/min. *Liver International.* 2016;36(6): 798-801.
[33] Saxena V, Koraishy FM, Sise ME, Lim JK, Schmidt M, Chung RT, et al. Safety and efficacy of sofosbuvir-containing regimens in hepatitis C-infected patients with impaired renal function. *Liver international: official journal of the International Association for the Study of the Liver.* 2016;36(6):807-16.
[34] Colombo M, Aghemo A, Liu H, Zhang J, Dvory-Sobol H, Hyland R, et al. Treatment with ledipasvir–sofosbuvir for 12 or 24 weeks in

kidney transplant recipients with chronic hepatitis C virus genotype 1 or 4 infection: a randomized trial. *Annals of internal medicine.* 2017;166(2):109-17.

[35] Reddy K, Sulkowski M, Hassan M, Levitsky J, O'Leary J, Brown R, et al. Safety and efficacy of new DAA regimens in kidney and liver transplant recipients with hepatitis C: interval results from the HCV-target study. *Journal of Hepatology.* 2016;64(2):S783-S4.

[36] Beste LA, Green PK, Berry K, Kogut MJ, Allison SK, Ioannou GN. Reply to: "Direct-acting antiviral therapy in patients with hepatocellular cancer: The timing of treatment is everything" and "More extended indication of DAA therapy in patients with HCC, affordability, and further statistical considerations." *Journal of hepatology.* 2017.

[37] Cortesi PA, Belli LS, Facchetti R, Mazzarelli C, Perricone G, De Nicola S, et al. The optimal timing of hepatitis C therapy in liver transplant-eligible patients: Cost-effectiveness analysis of new opportunities. *Journal of viral hepatitis.* 2018;25(7):791-801.

[38] Mogalian E, German P, Kearney BP, Yang CY, Brainard D, McNally J, et al. Use of multiple probes to assess transporter-and cytochrome P450-mediated drug–drug interaction potential of the pangenotypic HCV NS5A inhibitor velpatasvir. *Clinical pharmacokinetics.* 2016;55(5):605-13.

[39] Ly KN, Jiles RB, Teshale EH, Foster MA, Pesano RL, Holmberg SD. Hepatitis C virus infection among reproductive-aged women and children in the United States, 2006 to 2014. *Annals of internal medicine.* 2017;166(11):775-82.

[40] Koneru A. Increased hepatitis C virus (HCV) detection in women of childbearing age and potential risk for vertical transmission—United States and Kentucky, 2011–2014. *MMWR Morbidity and mortality weekly report.* 2016;65.

[41] *HCV in pregnancy 2019* [Available from https://www.hcvguidelines.org/unique-populations/pregnancy.

[42] Registry RP. *FDA Pregnancy list* [Available from http://www.ribavirinpregnancyregistry.com/.

In: The Pharmacological Guide to Sofosbuvir ISBN: 978-1-53616-476-3
Editor: Vijay Gayam   © 2019 Nova Science Publishers, Inc.

Chapter 5

MANAGEMENT OF PATIENTS CO-INFECTED WITH HCV/HIV AND HCV/HBV

Amrendra Kumar Mandal[1,*], Jasdeep Singh Sidhu[1], Benjamin Tiongson[1], Pavani Garlapati[1], Pallav Patel[2] and Vijay Gayam[1]

[1] Department of Internal Medicine, Interfaith Medical Center
Brooklyn, NY, US

[2] Department of Internal Medicine, Kaweah Delta Medical Center
Visalia, CA, US

ABSTRACT

The treatment of hepatitis C virus co-infections remains complex. Fortunately, new studies have revealed encouraging new regimens in the treatment of patients co-infected with Human immunodeficiency or Hepatitis B Viruses. Like Hepatitis B, C and, Human immunodeficiency viruses share similar routes of transmission, the likelihood of increased morbidity and mortality for any number of complications arising from these conditions remain significant. Furthermore, co-infection leads to

---

[*] Corresponding Author's E-mail: Amandal@interfaithmedical.com.

serious livers problems arising from more aggressive liver disease, advancing fibrosis, and earlier progression to end-stage liver disease. Therefore, eradication of Hepatitis C virus in co-infected patients remains a priority to achieve an overall improvement of public health. The recent development of new sofosbuvir-based direct-acting antivirals for the treatment of Hepatitis C virus has displayed excellent results in terms of sustained virologic response. However, treatment of Hepatitis C virus co-infections remains a challenge, owing to the possibility of drug-drug interactions, high rates of adverse events, increased pill burden, and lengthy treatment durations. Furthermore, there is also a risk of reactivation of HBV infection with the use of direct-acting antivirals. Thus, appropriate strategies should be employed in the treatment of Hepatitis C virus and its co-infections.

Keywords: chronic hepatitis C, hepatitis B virus, direct-acting antiviral agents, sustained virologic response, human immunodeficiency virus

ABBREVIATIONS

HCV	Hepatitis C virus
HIV	Human Immunodeficiency Virus
HBV	Hepatitis B virus
DAA	Direct acting antivirals
ART	Anti-retroviral therapy
SVR	Sustained virologic response
GFR	Glomerular Filtration Rate
TAF	Tenofovir alafenamide
TDF	Tenofovir disoproxil fumarate
SOF	sofosbuvir
CHB	Chronic hepatitis B
ALT	Alanine aminotransferase
AASLD	American Association for the Study of Liver Diseases

1. INTRODUCTION

There is an estimated 4 to 5 million people chronically infected with both human immunodeficiency virus (HIV) type 1 and hepatitis C virus (HCV) infection worldwide [1]. HCV infection is a leading cause of death in individuals infected with HIV, as HCV-related liver disease is progressed by HIV. Furthermore, HIV/HCV co-infected patients suffer from more liver-related morbidity and mortality, non-hepatic organ dysfunction, and overall mortality than HCV-mono-infected patients [2, 3]. Even in the era of effective HIV antiretroviral therapy, HIV infection remains independently associated with advanced liver fibrosis and cirrhosis in patients with HIV/HCV co-infection [4-7]. Therefore, appropriate management of both diseases is pivotal to prevent liver-related morbidity and mortality in this population. In a recent meta-analysis of HCV/HIV co-infected treated patients, it was found that in addition to maintenance of HIV viral suppression, there is also a small rise in CD4 count as compared with HIV mono-infected patients [8].

Current guidelines indicate direct-acting antivirals (DAA) regimens as the therapy of choice for both HCV and HCV/HIV co-infection. These agents target one of the non-structural proteins–NS3/4A protease, NS5B polymerase, and the NS5A protein–critically involved in HCV replication. Clinical trials have revealed comparable efficacy with DAA regimens in both HCV mono-infection and HCV/HIV co-infection [9, 10]. However, significant drug interaction between DAA and anti-retroviral therapy (ART) is a primary concern for therapy in HCV/HIV co-infected groups [11]. Sofosbuvir, an oral nucleotide analog inhibitor of the HCV non-structural 5B (NS5B) polymerase, has recently been approved for the treatment of patients across all HCV infected genotypes [12]. Among DAA regimens, sofosbuvir has minimal drug interactions with ART, supporting the use of sofosbuvir in combination with ART and other DAAs for the treatment of HCV/HIV co-infected patients.

The SVR rates in several clinical trials, where various regimens including ledipasvir/sofosbuvir, daclatasvir plus sofosbuvir, sofosbuvir/ velpatasvir, glecaprevir/pibrentasvir were used, ranged from 95% to 98%, which is similar to those in patients with HCV mono-infection [13-16]. However, there are few real-world clinical studies that have shown mixed sustained virologic response (SVR) in HCV/HIV co-infection.

Although, it has been shown that other unique HCV infected populations (e.g., co-morbid substance abusers) have had encouraging results in achieving overall SVR 12 (94.8%) [17].

1.1. Treatment of Patients in HCV/HIV Co-Infection

A new era of interferon-free HCV treatment has begun and is efficacious even in patients with HCV/HIV co-infection. However, there have been mixed reports of real-world efficacy in published literature. In a prospective study also from Spain reported a total of 1,634 participants; 1,152 (70%) were HCV-mono-infected patients and 482 (30%) HCV/HIV-co-infected patients. Both the groups, including mono-infected and co-infected patients, had SVR12 rates of 97% and 94% respectively. There was no difference in SVR12 rates between two these two groups even on subgroup analysis for cirrhosis, genotype, and DAA combination [18]. This was identical to another real-world study conducted by Gayam et al., the efficacy and tolerability of DAAs were retrospectively analyzed in HCV/HIV co-infection patients (n = 74) compared with (n = 253) with HCV mono-infection. The overall SVR rate in the entire cohort was 94%, although SVR rates were found to be higher in HCV mono-infected patients compared to those with HCV/HIV co-infection (96% vs. 86%, p = 0.005). In multivariate regression analysis, HIV positive groups were the only one found to be an independent factor in predicting treatment response; HIV viral load and CD4 cell count was not found to affect SVR12 rates. The study population was mostly African Americans, representing 64.5% of the entire cohort [19]. Furthermore, there were 68 (20.8%) patients with previous exposure to treatment, and the most common HCV genotype was 1a for both groups (62.2% in co-infection vs. 53.4% in mono-infection), with the comparable proportion of patients with compensated cirrhosis (14% vs. 23%, p = 0.103). Unlike in clinical trials, some co-infected patients had detectable HIV RNA in the blood. Lastly, the authors of this study also found that HCV/HIV co-infected patients had similar adverse event profiles when compared to HCV mono-infected patients. Both had anemia and leukopenia as common adverse events, which is consistent with the results of prior studies [19].

In contrast to the study above, SVR12 rates in patients with HIV co-infection who were treated with DAAs were only 86.3% (221/256 patients), which is significantly lower than 94.9% (205/216) in patients with HCV mono-infection treated with DAAs ($p = 0.002$). Moreover, HIV infection was found to be an independent predictor of failure to achieve SVR12 in multivariate logistic regression analysis. However, it was reported that about one half (n = 108/256, 42%) of the HCV/HIV co-infected patients were treated with simeprevir + sofosbuvir, could have resulted in treatment failure [16].

Therefore, it is yet an unsolved issue whether the response to DAAs in HCV/HIV co-infected patients is worse than in HCV mono-infected patients in the real world. Although most recent studies are leaning towards a comparable efficacy, as evidenced by large multi-center prospective studies (e.g., German hepatitis C cohort- GECCO-1, ANRS CO13-HEPAVIH cohort) [20, 21].

In clinical trials with a strict pre-defined design, there is no difference in SVR rates between co-infected and mono-infected patients. Liver disease progression should be monitored at regular intervals in case HCV treatment is delayed for any reason. HIV/HCV-co-infected patients should be continuously monitored, and physicians should pay attention to the complex drug-drug interactions that can occur between DAAs and ART. Further studies to investigate the efficacy of DAA regimens can be done, but healthcare policy should still be directed to treat all patients in this unique population, as the morbidity and mortality benefit of treatment remains significant. Many barriers to HCV therapy have been addressed with the development of DAA regimens, and thus, its use should still be advocated [10, 13, 22]. Similar to HCV-mono-infected patients, HIV/HCV-co-infected patients cured with peg-interferon/ribavirin have lower rates of hepatic decompensation, hepatocellular carcinoma, and liver-related mortality [18, 23].

Table 1 showed a summary of drug interactions with DAAs and ART. Drug interaction can be accessed at the US Department of Health and Human Services HIV treatment guidelines (https://aidsinfo.nih.gov/guidelines) and the University of Liverpool website (www.hep-druginteractions.org).

2. SOFOSBUVIR CONTAINING REGIMENS FOR HCV/HIV CO-INFECTION

Several treatment regimens are summarized in Table 1.

Table 1. Sofosbuvir-based regimens for the treatment of HCV with HIV co-infection

Regimen	Duration
Daclatasvir 60mg + Sofosbuvir 400mg	Once a day for 12 weeks
Simeprevir 150mg + Sofosbuvir 400mg	Once a day for 12 weeks
Ledipasvir 100mg/Sofosbuvir 400mg	Once a day for 12 weeks
Sofosbuvir 400mg/Velpatasvir 100mg/Voxilaprevir 100mg	Once a day for 12 weeks

2.1. Daclatasvir + Sofosbuvir

In the ALLY-3 clinical trial, Wyles et al. evaluated the 12-week regimen of daclatasvir plus sofosbuvir in patients with HIV/HCV co-infection [14]. In this open-label clinical trial, treatment-naive and -experienced HIV/HCV-co-infected patients received once-daily daclatasvir (60 mg dose) and sofosbuvir (400 mg), while treatment for HIV mostly used ritonavir-boosted darunavir, atazanavir, or lopinavir, efavirenz, nevirapine, rilpivirine, raltegravir, and dolutegravir. The combination of daclatasvir and sofosbuvir once daily for 12 weeks achieved SVR12 in 97% of HIV/HCV-co-infected patients across all genotype infection and was safe and well-tolerated. Ninety-seven percent of treatment-naive patients and 98% of treatment-experienced patients achieved SVR. It was also observed that the eight weeks regimen had a lower SVR rate. Factors associated with relapse in this patient group included high baseline HCV RNA level (>2 million IU/mL; 69%), concomitant use of a boosted darunavir-based antiretroviral regimen with 30 mg of daclatasvir (67%), and the presence of compensated cirrhosis (60%) [14].

2.1.1. Pharmacology and Drug Interaction Data

Daclatasvir had cytochrome P450 (CYP) 3A4 related metabolism and is therefore vulnerable to drug-drug interactions with potent inducers and inhibitors of this enzyme. In this case, daclatasvir must be increased from 60 mg to 90 mg when used with efavirenz, etravirine, or nevirapine [24]. Furthermore, the dosage should be decreased from 60 mg to 30 mg when used with ritonavir-boosted atazanavir, cobicistat-boosted atazanavir, or elvitegravir/cobicistat [25].

However, daclatasvir dose of 60 mg should be used with ritonavir-boosted darunavir and ritonavir-boosted lopinavir.

2.2. Ledipasvir/Sofosbuvir

In the phase 2 ERADICATE trial, safety and efficacy were assessed for 12 weeks of ledipasvir/sofosbuvir on HCV genotype 1 patients who were treatment naïve and without cirrhosis. Although the inclusion criteria for patients receiving antiretroviral therapy allowed CD4 cell counts > 100/mm^3, the median CD4 cell count was 576/mm^3. Overall, 98% achieved SVR12, (n = 13/13, 100%) in the treatment-naive arm and (n = 36/37, 97.3%) in the treatment-experienced arm). Renal function was monitored at regular intervals during this trial and after administration of study drugs with the relevant labs. No clinically significant changes in these parameters or renal toxicity were observed [9].

Another large trial, ION-4, also reported similar outcomes with ledipasvir/sofosbuvir. A total of 335 HCV treatment-naive and -

experienced HIV/HCV-co-infected patients were enrolled in the study and received ledipasvir/sofosbuvir once daily for 12 weeks. Patients received tenofovir disoproxil fumarate (TDF) and emtricitabine with raltegravir (44%), efavirenz (48%), or rilpivirine (9%). The overall SVR12 rate was 96% (321/335). Monitoring of renal function was done due to modest increases in TDF levels for those patients taking combination ledipasvir/sofosbuvir with tenofovir and a non-nucleoside reverse transcriptase-based regimens. Only one patient discontinued tenofovir treatment due to a worsening renal function suggestive of renal tubular disease, although this improved after switching to efavirenz/raltegravir and renally dosed emtricitabine [13].

Neither the ERADICATE nor the ION-4 study investigators reported clinically significant changes in CD4 cell counts or HIV RNA levels in the study participants. Thus, these data suggest that 12 weeks of ledipasvir/sofosbuvir is a safe and effective regimen for HIV/HCV-co-infected patients with genotype 1 infection taking selected antiretroviral therapy. A shorter course of 8 weeks is not recommended due to lower SVR rates demonstrated in trials [26].

2.2.1. Pharmacology and Drug Interaction Data

Drug interaction studies of ledipasvir (with or without sofosbuvir) with antiretroviral drugs in uninfected persons did not identify clinically significant interactions with abacavir, dolutegravir, emtricitabine, lamivudine, raltegravir, or rilpivirine [27]. Interactions with maraviroc and enfuvirtide are not expected based on their pharmacologic profiles. Ledipasvir's area under the curve (AUC) is decreased by 34% when co-administered with efavirenz-containing regimens and increased by 96% when co-administered with ritonavir-boosted atazanavir [28]. No dose adjustments of ledipasvir are recommended to account for these interactions.

Ledipasvir/sofosbuvir increases tenofovir levels when given as TDF, which may increase the risk of tenofovir-associated renal toxicity in combination with efavirenz, rilpivirine, dolutegravir, ritonavir-boosted atazanavir, or ritonavir-boosted darunavir. This combination should be avoided in patients with an estimated glomerular filtration rate (eGFR) <60 mL/min [28]. The absolute tenofovir levels are highest, and may exceed exposures for which there are established renal safety data, happens when TDF is administered with ritonavir- or cobicistat-containing regimens. Due to lack of sufficient safety data with this drug combination, consideration should be given to changing the antiretroviral regimen. TAF may be an alternative to TDF during ledipasvir/sofosbuvir treatment for patients who take cobicistat or ritonavir as part of their antiretroviral therapy.

In patients with an eGFR < 60 mL/min who are taking TDF with ledipasvir/sofosbuvir, renal parameters should be checked at baseline and the end of treatment. The lab parameters at baseline should include creatinine level, electrolytes, and urinary protein and glucose, according to recent guidelines for the management of chronic kidney disease in those with HIV [29]. ART should be switched for those at high risk for renal toxicity especially those with an eGFR between 30 mL/min and 60 mL/min or who have a preexisting likelihood of Fanconi syndrome, especially for patients using TDF and a ritonavir- or cobicistat-containing regimen. TDF should also be properly dosed and adjusted for eGFR at baseline and while on therapy [29].

2.3. Simeprevir /Sofosbuvir

The combination of simeprevir plus sofosbuvir, with or without ribavirin, was evaluated in the phase 2 COSMOS trial in patients with HCV mono-infection [30]. This study is the main basis for the recommendation supporting the use of this combination for genotype 1a or 1b mono-infection. Simeprevir plus sofosbuvir has been used anecdotally in patients with HIV/HCV co-infection, with a recent report of achieving SVR in 92% (11/12) of patients [31].

2.3.1. Pharmacology and Drug Interaction Data

Metabolism of simeprevir is typically by CYP3A4 and is therefore susceptible to drug interactions with inhibitors and inducers of this enzyme. Simeprevir is also an inhibitor of OATP1B1 and P-gp. Drug interaction studies with antiretroviral drugs in HIV-uninfected volunteers suggest no substantial interactions with tenofovir, rilpivirine, dolutegravir, or raltegravir. However, simeprevir concentrations were substantially decreased when dosed with efavirenz and substantially increased when dosed with ritonavir-boosted darunavir [32]. However, the use with efavirenz, etravirine, cobicistat, or boosted HIV protease inhibitors are not recommended [33].

2.4. Sofosbuvir/Velpatasvir

The safety and efficacy of 12 weeks of sofosbuvir/velpatasvir were evaluated in a phase 3 study among 106 antiretroviral-controlled, HIV/HCV-co-infected patients. All genotypes were enrolled in the study, and 18% of the patients had compensated cirrhosis. HIV was controlled on ART including non-nucleoside reverse-transcriptase inhibitor- (rilpivirine), integrase inhibitor- (raltegravir or elvitegravir/cobicistat), or ritonavir-boosted protease inhibitor- (atazanavir, lopinavir, or darunavir) based regimens with either tenofovir/emtricitabine or abacavir/lamivudine. Fifty-three percent (56/106) of participants were on TDF with a pharmacologic boosting agent (either ritonavir or cobicistat) [22]. SVR12 was 95% with 2 relapses, both occurring in genotype 1a-infected patients. Similar results were noted in patients with compensated cirrhosis and those with baseline NS5A RASs (n = 12 at 15% threshold; SVR12 = 100%). There were no clinically significant changes in serum creatinine or eGFR, and no patients required a change in their antiretroviral therapy during the study period [22].

In general, few HIV/HCV-co-infected patients with compensated cirrhosis have been included in clinical trials of DAAs, and no data are available regarding HIV/HCV-co-infected patients with renal insufficiency or who have undergone solid organ transplantation. Despite a lack of data, it is highly likely that response rates are similar to those of HCV-mono-infected patients, as no study to date in the DAA era has shown a lower efficacy for HIV/HCV-co-infected patients. Therefore, the proper guidance should be used if treatment is warranted with consideration for any drug interactions.

2.4.1. Pharmacology and Drug Interaction Data

Velpatasvir is available only in a fixed-dose combination tablet with sofosbuvir. Velpatasvir is metabolized by CYP3A4, CYP2C8, and CYP2B6. It does not appear to inhibit or induce any CYP enzymes. Velpatasvir is a substrate for P-gp and BCRP, and inhibits P-gp, BCRP, and OATP1B1/1B3 but does not induce any transporters. In patients with an eGFR < 60 mL/min, consider the use of TAF instead of TDF in those requiring ritonavir- or cobicistat-containing antiretroviral therapy. If the combination TDF with a ritonavir- or cobicistat-containing antiretroviral therapy is required in patients with an eGFR < 60 mL/min, renal parameters should be checked at baseline and regularly after that while on sofosbuvir/velpatasvir [34].

Velpatasvir exposures are significantly reduced with efavirenz, and this combination is not recommended [34]. Etravirine has not been studied with sofosbuvir/velpatasvir and is also not recommended [34]. Indirect bilirubin level increases have been reported when sofosbuvir/velpatasvir was used in patients on atazanavir/ritonavir [34].

TAF may be an alternative to TDF, as shown in healthy volunteers during sofosbuvir/velpatasvir treatment for patients who take cobicistat or ritonavir as part of their antiretroviral therapy [35]. However, there are no safety data for this combination in HIV/HCV-co-infected patients.

2.5. Sofosbuvir/Velpatasvir/Voxilaprevir

There is no data for the treatment of HIV/HCV-co-infected patients with Sofosbuvir/Velpatasvir/Voxilaprevir. Despite a lack of data, it is highly likely that response rates in HIV/HCV-co-infected patients will be similar to those of HCV-mono-infected patients, as no study to date in the DAA era has shown a lower efficacy for HIV/HCV-co-infected patients.

Therefore, the guidelines above should be followed, with the consideration of drug-drug interactions.

2.5.1. Pharmacology and Drug Interaction Data

Voxilaprevir is a substrate for P-gp, OATP, BCRP, CYP3A, CYP1A2, and CYP2C8. Voxilaprevir inhibits OATP, P-gp, and BCRP. Voxilaprevir AUC is increased by 331% with ritonavir-boosted atazanavir, and this combination is not recommended [24]. Voxilaprevir AUC is increased 171% with tenofovir alafenamide/emtricitabine/elvitegravir/cobicistat, and 143% with tenofovir disoproxil fumarate/emtricitabine and ritonavir-boosted darunavir. Although these increases in voxilaprevir AUC were not clinically relevant by the manufacturer or the United States Food and Drug Association, due to lack of clinical safety data, close monitoring for hepatic toxicity is recommended until additional safety data are available in HIV/HCV-co-infected patients. The liver enzyme is recommended testing every 4 weeks [35].

Table 2. Guidelines for Treatment of Patients with HBV and HCV co-infection

All HBsAg-positive patients should be tested for HCV infection using the anti-HCV test
DAA should be recommended for patients with detection in viral load [45].
HBV treatment should be based on HBV-DNA and ALT levels as per the American Association for the study of Liver Disease (AASLD) guidelines for mono-infected patients [46].
HBsAg-positive patients are at risk of HBV-DNA and ALT flares with HCV DAA therapy, and monitoring of HBV DNA levels every 4-8 weeks during treatment and for three months post-treatment is indicated in those who do not meet treatment criteria for mono-infected patients per the AASLD HBV guidelines [44].
HBsAg-negative, anti-HBc–positive patients with HCV are at very low risk of reactivation with HCV-DAA therapy. ALT levels should be monitored at baseline, at the end of treatment, and during follow-up, with HBV-DNA and HBsAg testing reserved for those whose ALT levels increase or fail to normalize during treatment or post-treatment [44].

Velpatasvir absorption is pH-dependent and its AUC is reduced by approximately 50% when given with omeprazole 20 mg daily as part of the fixed-dose sofosbuvir/velpatasvir/voxilaprevir combination. Real-world retrospective studies by Gayam et al. have shown that patient has tolerated

DAA treatment regimens, with patient's high treatment adherence [17, 36-38].

3. MANAGEMENT OF HCV/HBV CO-INFECTION

The treatment goals for the management of HCV/HBV are the same as with any patient with chronic hepatitis B (CHB). Treatment goals are to reduce the risk of progression to cirrhosis and further complications such as decompensation and hepatocellular carcinoma. In HBV-HCV–co-infected patients, HCV-RNA and HBV-DNA levels reflect viral activity, responsible for related liver complications. In the case of detectable HCV RNA, HCV treatment should be initiated; the same goes for cases of hepatitis B infections if HBV DNA is detectable. There is an interesting observation that treatment of CHB or HBV infections may alter the activity of the other virus, and therefore monitoring of lab parameters during and after therapy should be followed to assess for viral activity and after that, treatment as indicated [39].

Previously, in the interferon era, the treatment of choice for patients co-infected with HBV and HCV infections was pegylated-interferon and ribavirin for 24-48 weeks (based on HCV genotype). Moderate-to-high rates of HCV eradication and HBV suppression were reported with this combination [40, 41]. However, a rebound in serum HBV DNA after an initial decline and increased HBV replication in patients with undetectable HBV DNA before treatment have been reported with peg-interferon and ribavirin [42]. Similarly, DAA for HCV therapy has been reported to increase HBV-DNA levels in HBsAg-positive patients and to elevate alanine aminotransferase concurrently with HBV reactivation. Despite these events, the progression of liver decompensation and liver failure are very low [43]. The majority of reported reactivation events (elevated alanine aminotransferase with elevated HBV DNA) occurred between 4 and 12 weeks of DAA treatment [3]. In HBV-HCV–co-infected patients with cirrhosis or those fulfilling recommended criteria for HBV treatment, antiviral therapy for HBV should be started concurrently with DAA therapy. The antivirals used for HBV infections are entecavir, TDF, or TAF. In chronic HCV infection having HBsAg-negative, anti-HBc–positive, monitoring alanine aminotransferase levels are useful, along with HBV DNA levels. There are no known interactions between HBV antivirals (entecavir, TDF, or TAF) and approved HCV DAAs [44].

For triply infected patients with HIV, HBV, and HCV, TDF/TAF is recommended as it is used for HBV and also included in the treatment regimen for HIV infections [44]. The use of ART before initiation of HCV or HBV therapy should be carefully understood.

4. Measures to Improve Treatment Compliance

Increased adherence to DAAs, ARTs, and antiviral for HBV infections are associated with high SVR rates. On the other hand, non-adherence to therapy is linked with a risk of virological breakthrough or post-treatment relapse. Measures to increase compliance include an interdisciplinary approach, which includes access to a multidisciplinary team consisting of a clinician, nursing clinical assessment and monitoring, virology, drug and alcohol services, Infectious disease specialist, psychiatrist support for selected cases [47, 48]. To maximize the likelihood of benefit for patients who begin new HCV treatment regimens, especially for co-infections with HIV or HBV or combinations of all; resources should be devoted to patient pre-treatment assessment and preparation [49].

Conclusion

There are shared modes of transmission for HCV, HBV, and HIV infections with complex drug-drug interaction requiring DAA and ART to be used with consideration of its interaction. However, with the advent of newer DAAs, the efficacy of treatment for HCV/HIV co-infection has increased, as evidenced in recent clinical trials. Furthermore, real-world studies have also been encouraging for both HCV mono-infection and

HCV/HIV co-infection. Reactivation of HBV has been reported in patients starting DAA HCV therapy who are not on active HBV agents. Consistent with general recommendations for the assessment of both HIV- and HCV-infected patients, all patients initiating HCV DAA therapy should be assessed for HBV co-infection with HBsAg, anti-HBs, and anti-HBc testing. However, there is no significant drug interaction between DAAs and HBV antivirals.

REFERENCES

[1] Balogun, MA; et al., The prevalence of hepatitis C in England and Wales. *J Infect*, 2002, 45(4), p. 219-26.

[2] De Re, V; et al., Impact of immunogenetic IL28B polymorphism on natural outcome of HCV infection. *Biomed Res Int*, 2014, **2014**, p. 710642.

[3] Chen, KX; Njoroge, FG. A review of HCV protease inhibitors. *Curr Opin Investig Drugs*, 2009, **10**(8), p. 821-37.

[4] Thein, HH; et al., Natural history of hepatitis C virus infection in HIV-infected individuals and the impact of HIV in the era of highly active antiretroviral therapy: a meta-analysis. *AIDS*, 2008, **22**(15), p. 1979-91.

[5] de Ledinghen, V; et al., Liver fibrosis on account of chronic hepatitis C is more severe in HIV-positive than HIV-negative patients despite antiretroviral therapy. *J Viral Hepat*, 2008, **15**(6), p. 427-33.

[6] Fierer, DS; et al., Rapid progression to decompensated cirrhosis, liver transplant, and death in HIV-infected men after primary hepatitis C virus infection. *Clin Infect Dis*, 2013, **56**(7), p. 1038-43.

[7] Kirk, GD; et al., HIV, age, and the severity of hepatitis C virus-related liver disease: a cohort study. *Ann Intern Med*, 2013, **158**(9), p. 658-66.

[8] Martin, TC; et al., Hepatitis C virus reinfection incidence and treatment outcome among HIV-positive MSM. *AIDS*, 2013, **27**(16), p. 2551-7.

[9] Osinusi, A; et al., Virologic response following combined ledipasvir and sofosbuvir administration in patients with HCV genotype 1 and HIV co-infection. *JAMA*, 2015, **313**(12), p. 1232-9.

[10] Bhattacharya, D; et al., Effectiveness of All-Oral Antiviral Regimens in 996 Human Immunodeficiency Virus/Hepatitis C Virus Genotype 1-Coinfected Patients Treated in Routine Practice. *Clin Infect Dis*, 2017, **64**(12), p. 1711-1720.

[11] Khatri, A; et al., Evaluation of Drug-Drug Interactions between Direct-Acting Anti-Hepatitis C Virus Combination Regimens and the HIV-1 Antiretroviral Agents Raltegravir, Tenofovir, Emtricitabine, Efavirenz, and Rilpivirine. *Antimicrob Agents Chemother*, 2016, **60**(5), p. 2965-71.

[12] Welzel, TM; et al., Ombitasvir, paritaprevir, and ritonavir plus dasabuvir for 8 weeks in previously untreated patients with hepatitis C virus genotype 1b infection without cirrhosis (GARNET): a single-arm, open-label, phase 3b trial. *Lancet Gastroenterol Hepatol*, 2017, **2**(7), p. 494-500.

[13] Naggie, S; et al., Ledipasvir and Sofosbuvir for HCV in Patients Coinfected with HIV-1. *N Engl J Med*, 2015, **373**(8), p. 705-13.

[14] Wyles, DL; et al., Daclatasvir plus Sofosbuvir for HCV in Patients Coinfected with HIV-1. *N Engl J Med*, 2015, **373**(8), p. 714-25.

[15] Rockstroh, JK; et al., Efficacy and Safety of Glecaprevir/Pibrentasvir in Patients Coinfected With Hepatitis C Virus and Human Immunodeficiency Virus Type 1: The EXPEDITION-2 Study. *Clin Infect Dis*, 2018, **67**(7), p. 1010-1017.

[16] Neukam, K; et al., HIV-coinfected patients respond worse to direct-acting antiviral-based therapy against chronic hepatitis C in real life than HCV-monoinfected individuals: a prospective cohort study. *HIV Clin Trials*, 2017, **18**(3), p. 126-134.

[17] Gayam, V; et al., Real-world study of hepatitis C treatment with direct-acting antivirals in patients with drug abuse and opioid agonist therapy. *Scand J Gastroenterol*, 2019, **54**(5), p. 646-655.

[18] Montes, ML; et al., Similar effectiveness of direct-acting antiviral against hepatitis C virus in patients with and without HIV infection. *AIDS*, 2017, **31**(9), p. 1253-1260.

[19] Gayam, V; et al., Real-World Clinical Efficacy and Tolerability of Direct-Acting Antivirals in Hepatitis C Monoinfection Compared to Hepatitis C/Human Immunodeficiency Virus Coinfection in a Community Care Setting. *Gut Liver*, 2018, **12**(6), p. 694-703.

[20] Sogni, P; et al., All-oral Direct-acting Antiviral Regimens in HIV/Hepatitis C Virus-coinfected Patients with Cirrhosis Are Efficient and Safe: Real-life Results from the Prospective ANRS CO13-HEPAVIH Cohort. *Clin Infect Dis*, 2016, **63**(6), p. 763-770.

[21] Ingiliz, P; et al., Sofosbuvir and Ledipasvir for 8 Weeks for the Treatment of Chronic Hepatitis C Virus (HCV) Infection in HCV-Monoinfected and HIV-HCV-Coinfected Individuals: Results from the German Hepatitis C Cohort (GECCO-01). *Clin Infect Dis*, 2016, **63**(10), p. 1320-1324.

[22] Wyles, D; et al., Sofosbuvir and Velpatasvir for the Treatment of Hepatitis C Virus in Patients Coinfected With Human Immunodeficiency Virus Type 1: An Open-Label, Phase 3 Study. *Clin Infect Dis*, 2017, **65**(1), p. 6-12.

[23] Berenguer, J; et al., Sustained virological response to interferon plus ribavirin reduces liver-related complications and mortality in patients coinfected with human immunodeficiency virus and hepatitis C virus. *Hepatology*, 2009, **50**(2), p. 407-13.

[24] Bifano, M; et al., Assessment of pharmacokinetic interactions of the HCV NS5A replication complex inhibitor daclatasvir with antiretroviral agents: ritonavir-boosted atazanavir, efavirenz and tenofovir. *Antivir Ther*, 2013, **18**(7), p. 931-40.

[25] Smolders, EJ; et al., Management of drug interactions with direct-acting antivirals in Dutch HIV/hepatitis C virus-coinfected patients: adequate but not perfect. *HIV Med*, 2018, **19**(3), p. 216-226.

[26] Luetkemeyer, AF; et al., 12 Weeks of Daclatasvir in Combination with Sofosbuvir for HIV-HCV Coinfection (ALLY-2 Study):

Efficacy and Safety by HIV Combination Antiretroviral Regimens. *Clin Infect Dis*, 2016, **62**(12), p. 1489-96.

[27] Garrison, KL; et al., Drug-drug interaction profile of sofosbuvir/velpatasvir/voxilaprevir fixed-dose combination. *Journal of Hepatology*, 2017, **66**(1), p. S492-S493.

[28] German, P; et al., Drug interactions between direct acting anti-HCV antivirals sofosbuvir and ledipasvir and HIV antiretrovirals. *15th International Workshop on Clinical Pharmacology of HIV and Hepatitis Therapy*, 2014.

[29] Lucas, GM; et al., Clinical practice guideline for the management of chronic kidney disease in patients infected with HIV: 2014 update by the HIV Medicine Association of the Infectious Diseases Society of America. *Clin Infect Dis*, 2014, **59**(9), p. e96-138.

[30] Lawitz, E; et al., Sofosbuvir for previously untreated chronic hepatitis C infection. *N Engl J Med*, 2013, **368**(20), p. 1878-87.

[31] Del Bello, D; et al., Real-World Sustained Virologic Response Rates of Sofosbuvir-Containing Regimens in Patients Coinfected With Hepatitis C and HIV. *Clin Infect Dis*, 2016, **62**(12), p. 1497-1504.

[32] MacBrayne, CE; et al. Small increase in dolutegravir trough, but equivalent total exposure with simeprevir [P_48]. in *International Workshop on Clinical Pharmacology of Antiviral Therapy.*, June 14-16, 2017.

[33] Ouwerkerk-Mahadevan, S; et al., Drug-Drug Interactions with the NS3/4A Protease Inhibitor Simeprevir. *Clin Pharmacokinet*, 2016, **55**(2), p. 197-208.

[34] Disease, AAftSoL. *Pharmacology and Drug Interaction Data* [cited], 2019, Available from: https://www.hcvguidelines.org/unique-populations/hiv-hcv.

[35] Garrison, K; et al., *Drug-drug interaction profile of sofosbuvir/velpatasvir/voxilaprevir fixed-dose combination.*, 2017, **66**(1), p. S492-S493.

[36] Gayam, V; et al., Direct-Acting Antivirals in Chronic Hepatitis C Genotype 4 Infection in Community Care Setting. *Gastroenterology Res*, 2018, **11**(2), p. 130-137.

[37] Gayam, V; et al., Sofosbuvir Based Regimens in the Treatment of Chronic Hepatitis C with Compensated Liver Cirrhosis in Community Care Setting. *Int J Hepatol*, 2018, **2018**, p. 4136253.

[38] Gayam, V; et al., Sofosbuvir based regimens in the treatment of chronic hepatitis C genotype 1 infection in African-American patients: a community-based retrospective cohort study. *Eur J Gastroenterol Hepatol*, 2018, **30**(10), p. 1200-1207.

[39] Flisiak, R; et al., Recommendations for the treatment of hepatitis B in 2017. *Clin Exp Hepatol*, 2017, **3**(2), p. 35-46.

[40] Uyanikoglu, A; et al., Co-infection with hepatitis B does not alter treatment response in chronic hepatitis C. *Clin Res Hepatol Gastroenterol*, 2013, **37**(5), p. 485-90.

[41] Kim, YJ; et al., Clinical features and treatment efficacy of peginterferon alfa plus ribavirin in chronic hepatitis C patients coinfected with hepatitis B virus. *Korean J Hepatol*, 2011, **17**(3), p. 199-205.

[42] Potthoff, A; et al., The HEP-NET B/C co-infection trial: A prospective multicenter study to investigate the efficacy of pegylated interferon-alpha2b and ribavirin in patients with HBV/HCV co-infection. *J Hepatol*, 2008, **49**(5), p. 688-94.

[43] Belperio, PS; et al., Evaluation of hepatitis B reactivation among 62,920 veterans treated with oral hepatitis C antivirals. *Hepatology*, 2017, **66**(1), p. 27-36.

[44] Terrault, NA; et al., Update on prevention, diagnosis, and treatment of chronic hepatitis B: AASLD 2018 hepatitis B guidance. *Hepatology*, 2018, **67**(4), p. 1560-1599.

[45] Tseng, TC; Kao, JH. Clinical utility of quantitative HBsAg in natural history and nucleos(t)ide analogue treatment of chronic hepatitis B: new trick of old dog. *J Gastroenterol*, 2013, **48**(1), p. 13-21.

[46] Terrault, NA; et al., AASLD guidelines for treatment of chronic hepatitis B. *Hepatology*, 2016, **63**(1), p. 261-83.

[47] Dore, GJ; et al., Efficacy and safety of ombitasvir/paritaprevir/r and dasabuvir compared to IFN-containing regimens in genotype 1 HCV

patients: The MALACHITE-I/II trials. *J Hepatol*, 2016, **64**(1), p. 19-28.

[48] Alavian, SM; Aalaei-Andabili, SH. Education by a nurse increases the adherence to therapy in chronic hepatitis C patients. *Clin Gastroenterol Hepatol*, 2012, **10**(2), p. 203, author reply 203.

[49] Alexander, JA; et al., Patient-physician role relationships and patient activation among individuals with chronic illness. *Health Serv Res*, 2012, **47**(3 Pt 1), p. 1201-23.

In: The Pharmacological Guide to Sofosbuvir   ISBN: 978-1-53616-476-3
Editor: Vijay Gayam   © 2019 Nova Science Publishers, Inc.

Chapter 6

SOFOSBUVIR TREATMENT OF HEPATITIS C IN PEOPLE WITH PSYCHIATRIC ILLNESS AND SUBSTANCE USE DISORDERS

Benjamin Tiongson[1,]*, MD, Oluwole Jegede[1,†], MD, Olaniyi Olayinka[1,‡], MD, Pavani Garlapati[2,§], MD, Amrendra Kumar Mandal[2,||], MD, Vijay Gayam[2,¶], MD and Jason Hershberger[1,#], MD

[1]Department of Psychiatry and Behavioral Sciences, Interfaith Medical Center, Brooklyn, NY, US
[2]Department of Internal Medicine, Interfaith Medical Center, Brooklyn, NY, US

---

* Corresponding Author's E-mail: bctiongson@gmail.com.
† Author's E-mail: Ojegede@interfaithmedical.org.
‡ Author's E-mail: oolayinka@interfaithmedical.com.
§ Author's E-mail: docpavanireddy@gmail.com.
|| Author's E-mail: Amandal@interfaithmedical.com.
¶ Author's E-mail: vgayam@interfaithmedical.org.
# Author's E-mail: jhershberger@interfaithmedical.com.

ABSTRACT

There is a high comorbidity of chronic Hepatitis C among individuals with mental illness, particularly among the subpopulation of people who use drugs. Unfortunately, the undertreatment of Chronic Hepatitis C has contributed to a significant public health burden among people with mental illness. As in the general population, the natural history of Hepatitis C infection progression leads to chronic Hepatitis C and eventually cirrhosis, hepatic decompensation, and hepatocellular carcinoma. The introduction of direct-acting antiviral combinations has revolutionized the treatment of Chronic Hepatitis C virus infection. Compared to previous traditional interferon-based therapies, interferon-free oral direct-acting antiviral combinations with or without ribavirin have been shown to be superior in terms of reduced pill burden, ease of administration, safety and efficacy, regardless of these comorbidities. Sofosbuvir in combination with other direct-acting antivirals has emerged as the most promising drug in its class that came out the market, due to its activity against all genotypes, relatively safe adverse event profile and high success rates in achieving sustained virologic response. In this chapter, we will review the role of sofosbuvir in the treatment of chronic hepatitis C infection, with emphasis on people with comorbid mental illness and substance use disorders. We further reviewed recommendations for HCV testing and management of these populations as well as linkage to care strategies for these high-risk populations.

Keywords: sofosbuvir, direct-acting antivirals, sustained virologic response, Hepatitis C virus, substance use disorders, mental illness

ABBREVIATIONS

HCV	Hepatitis C Virus
CHC	Chronic Hepatitis C
IDU	Injection drug use
PWID	Persons who inject drugs
SMI	Serious Mental Illness
IFN	Interferon
RBV	Ribavirin
AE	Adverse Event

DAA	Direct-Acting Antivirals
SVR	Sustained Virologic Response
GT	Genotype
AASLD	American Association for the Study of Liver Disease
IDSA	Infectious Disease Society of America
EASL	European Association for the Study of Liver diseases
WHO	World Health Organization
INHSU	International Network on Hepatitis in Substance Users
OST	Opioid Substitution therapy
SOF	Sofosbuvir
FDA	Food and Drug Association
PWUD	Persons who use drugs
DCV	Daclatasvir
SMV	Simeprevir
BDI	Beck's Depression Inventory
LDV	Ledipasvir
RAV	Resistance Associated Variant
VEL	Velpatasvir
VOX	Voxilaprevir
PHQ 9	Patient Health Questionnaire 9
CDC	Centers for Disease Control
USPTSF	United States Preventive Services Task Force
STIRR	*Screen, Test, Immunize, Reduce risk, Refer*
MMTP	Methadone Maintenance Program

1. INTRODUCTION

Upon its discovery in 1989, Hepatitis C Virus (HCV) infection continues to be a global health burden, affecting an estimated 2.8% of the population, corresponding to >185 million worldwide [1]. Consequently, HCV-related diseases (e.g., cirrhosis and hepatocellular Carcinoma) from progression to Chronic Hepatitis C (CHC) have increased, reflecting the high incidence rates of hepatitis C during the mid-twentieth century from unregulated use of parenteral procedures and injection drug use (IDU) [2, 3]. The transmission of the virus is mainly through parenteral contact with contaminated body fluids, and the highest risk comes from Persons Who Inject Drugs (PWID), which is estimated to be 67% or 10 million of 16 million people in 148 countries positive for anti-HCV antibodies globally [2, 4-7]. This increased risk also holds true for patients with serious mental illness (SMI), albeit not to the same degree. In a meta-analysis conducted by Hughes et al., the pooled prevalence of HCV is also greater among persons with SMI, defined as a diagnosis of mental illness (e.g., schizophrenia, bipolar disorder, schizoaffective disorder or other psychoses) that is persistent, disabling, and requiring specialized psychiatric treatment as an outpatient or inpatient admission. They noted a prevalence as high as 17.4% compared to a 1% infection rate in the general population in North America alone [6]. Also, poor cultural and socioeconomic background predisposes to HCV infection [5, 8]. Among the population with the highest-burden are those with comorbid SMI and substance abuse history [5, 6, 9-11]. It is also reported that synergy within co-occurring infections or disorders increases the likelihood of transmission and progression of HCV, thus highlighting the significance of adequate screening of these populations, prevention, and treatment of these diseases and disorders [5].

The evolution of the standard of care was driven by the desire to reduce the public health burden and increase the efficacy and safety of CHC treatment. Previously, interferon (IFN)-based therapies caused undesirable side effects, which include IFN-induced bone marrow depression, flu-like symptoms, neuropsychiatric disorders, and autoimmune disorders. These side effects, along with the ribavirin (RBV)-induced hemolytic anemia, resulted in 10-20% premature withdrawals from IFN therapy overall, thus reducing adherence to therapy and discontinuation of treatment [12]. The shift of standard of care by pegylation of IFN improved efficiency and safety of the drug by increasing systemic retention, resulting in less need for frequent injections, but overall, adverse event (AE) profiles remain significant [13, 14]. The advent of first-generation direct-acting antivirals (DAA) marked the start of a highly specific treatment for CHC. These drugs targeting HCV NS3/4A serine protease (e.g., boceprevir, telaprevir) co-administered with pegylated-IFN and RBV increased sustained virologic response (SVR) rates when compared to peg-IFN and RBV alone, although its limited activity to other genotypes (GT) (except HCV GT1 infections), and severe adverse effects on patients with advanced disease (i.e., platelet count <100,000/mm^3, albumin <35 g/L) still represented a significant barrier to treatment [2, 15, 16]. Whereas the AE profile of IFN-based therapies prohibited treatment delivery to patients, another shift in the standard of care to newer second-generation IFN-free regimens consisting of combination DAAs has obviated the need for IFN and increased SVR rates overall [17, 18]. Favorable safety profiles decreased pill burden, treatment duration and increased adherence to treatment. It is also highly effective regardless of GT, prior treatment history, and cirrhosis status [19, 20].

Furthermore, these regimens have also been found to be effective and safe regardless of comorbid mental illness and substance use as evidenced in real-world studies [21-23]. In spite of these advancements, reluctance still exists in screening and treatment within these populations due to negative perceptions of persons who use drugs illicitly [2, 24-28]. Restrictions implemented by governments, based on fibrosis stage, recent drug use and prescriber type limit DAA therapy and is contradictory to local and international guidelines e.g., American Association for Study of Liver Diseases- Infectious Disease Society of America (AASLD-IDSA), European Association for the Study of Liver Disease (EASL), World Health Organization (WHO) and International Network on Hepatitis in Substance Users (INHSU), constituting a poor public health strategy [29]. In the US alone, 88% of US state Medicaid committees have issued restrictions to those who have a history of recent IDU, illicit drugs use or are receiving opioid substitution therapy (OST) [30]. Stringent eligibility criteria for DAA-based therapies, which include requirements for periods of abstinence and urine drug screening are inconsistent with recommendations by most professional organizations and limits treatment and consequently, adds to the public health burden.

Among the DAAs that came out of the market, sofosbuvir (SOF), an NS5B nucleotide polymerase inhibitor has emerged to be highly successful and is the most widely used drug in the treatment of HCV infection. Marketed through Gilead Science, SOF is a pro-drug metabolized thru the active ingredient uridine triphosphate (GS-461203) to inhibit the NS5B protein thru competitive inhibition, used by the virus as an RNA polymerase for replication [19]. The Food and Drug Association (FDA) have approved SOF in combination with other classes of DAA (e.g., NS5A inhibitors, NS3/4A protease inhibitors) with or without RBV for the treatment of CHC for all GTs [2, 19].

In this chapter, we will review the literature supporting the use of SOF in treating patients with CHC. Pivotal studies supporting the use of SOF will be highlighted. Evidenced-based public health strategies and recommendations for prevention and management of HCV infected person with comorbid substance use and mental illness will also be discussed.

2. CLINICAL EFFICACY AND SAFETY OF SOFOSBUVIR-BASED TREATMENTS

The goal of HCV therapy is the permanent eradication of the HCV and prevention of its associated complications. The standard efficacy endpoint of CHC treatment is through an SVR, defined as the absence of detectable HCV RNA viral load after 12-24 weeks of treatment. Limited safety and efficacy data exist on the use of DAA regimens for Persons Who Use Drugs (PWUD) and more so for the mental health population, and expert recommendations for pharmacologic treatment in these high-risk populations remains the same as the general population. More importantly, there is an increased emphasis on the identification and screening of these individuals to reduce the associated public health burden [5]. Pre- and post-marketing studies supporting the use of SOF combinations are presented in Table 1. Currently, the AASLD-IDSA has issued treatment guidelines recommending combination therapies using second-generation DAAs for the treatment of HCV infection. The recommended SOF-based combinations are presented in Table 2 [31]. The efficacy and safety of the different drug combinations are also discussed below.

2.1. Efficacy and Safety of Sofosbuvir and Daclatasvir Combination

Daclatasvir (DCV) is a pan-genotypic HCV NS5A replication complex inhibitor, and when combined with SOF, has potent antiviral activity and broad genotypic coverage [32]. In phase II open-label clinical trial conducted by Sulkowski et al., 88 treatment naïve patients with HCV GT 1, 2 or 3 received SOF 400 mg and DCV 60mg orally once a day, with or without RBV initially for 24 weeks. Additional 123 GT1 patients were later recruited with patients grouped to either being treatment naïve or had prior treatment failure. They received the same regimen of DCV and SOF with or without RBV for 12 weeks or 24 weeks, respectively. Overall SVR rate for GT1 at 12 weeks was 98% for both treatments naïve and those with prior protease inhibitor non-response. Ninety-two percent of GT2 patients and 89% of GT3 patients achieved SVR at week 12. Adjunction with RBV and SOF with a lead-in phase (1 week of SOF before 23 weeks of DCV+SOF) did not provide significant benefits. The group concluded that once-daily oral treatment with a combination of SOF+DCV with or without RBV had high rates of sustained virologic response in untreated patients with HCV GT 1,2,3. This is also the same for patients with GT1 infection with prior treatment failure with protease inhibitors. Most common AE reported was fatigue, headache, and nausea [32].

Clinical safety and efficacy were also evaluated in specific populations using DCV and SOF with transplant patients and HIV/HCV co-infected, respectively. ALLY-3 looked at the difficult to treat HCV GT 3 infected population (Table 1). In these trials, 12 weeks of SOF + DCV consistently reported high rates of SVR, regardless of previous HCV treatment, presence of cirrhosis, disease characteristics or demographics. Favorable safety profiles suggest higher utility in a broader range of patients, further supporting the use of this combination for all patients [33-35].

Table 1. Clinical efficacy and tolerability of Sofosbuvir-based combinations

Name/Treatment group, study type/year	Patient characteristics	Treatment groups	Duration of therapy	Overall SVR rate	Adverse Events (AE)
SOF+DCV, Phase II trial, (2014), [32]	Treatment naïve, Previously treated Genotype 1-3	Group A and B (n=31) SOF DCV+SOF Group C and D (n=28) DCV+SOF Group E and F (n=29) DCV+SOF+RBV Group G (n=41) DCV+SOF Group H (n=41) DCV+SOF+RBV Group I (n=21) DCV+SOF Group J (n=20) DCV+SOF+RBV	1 week 23 weeks 24 weeks 24 weeks 12 weeks 12 weeks 24 weeks 24 weeks	>90%	Fatigue, nausea, and headache [a]
ALLY-1, Phase III trial, 2015, [33]	Treatment naïve, Treatment-experienced, Cirrhosis (decompensated/ compensated), Post-liver transplant Genotype 1-4, 6	Advanced cirrhosis (n=60) Post-transplantation cohort (n=53)	12 weeks 12 weeks	80-100%	Headache, fatigue, anemia [a], One patient discontinued treatment due to Ribavirin-induced anemia
ALLY-2, phase III trial, 2015, [34]	203 HIV/HCV co-infected patients Genotype 1-4	DCV+SOF (treatment naïve, n=101) DCV+SOF (treatment naïve, n=50) DCV+SOF (treatment-experienced, n=52)	12 weeks 8 weeks 12 weeks	76-97%	No study discontinuation due to AEs

Name/Treatment group, study type/year	Patient characteristics	Treatment groups	Duration of therapy	Overall SVR rate	Adverse Events (AE)
ALLY-3, phase III clinical trial, 2015, [35]	152 treatment naïve, treatment-experienced Genotype 3	DCV+SOF (treatment naïve, n=101) DCV+SOF (treatment-experienced, n=51)	12 weeks 12 weeks	89%	Head, fatigue, and nausea [a]
Autorisation Temporaire d'Utilisation program/DCV+SOF+RBV Real-world study, 2017, [36]	407 HIV/HCV co-infected patients, Genotype 1,3 and 4 Advanced liver disease (F3, F4 fibrosis, and/or severe extra-hepatic HCV manifestation)	DCV+SOF (n=87) DCV+SOF+RBV (n=16) DCV+SOF (n=260) DCV+SOF+RBV (n=42)	12 weeks 12 weeks 24 weeks 24 weeks	92%	Seven discontinued treatment, 10 deaths, 3 of which is considered treatment-related
ELECTRON-2, phase II trial, 2014, [37]	113 treatment naïve and null-responders, Genotype 1	LDV/SOF+RBV (treatment naïve, n=25) LDV/SOF+RBV (prior null responders, n=9) SOF+GS9669+RBV (treatment naïve, n=25) SOF+GS9669+RBV (prior null responders, n=10) SOF/LDV+RBV (prior null responders with cirrhosis, n =9) SOF/LDV (prior null responders with cirrhosis, n=10) SOF/LDV+RBV (treatment naïve (n=25)	12 weeks 12 weeks 12 weeks 12 weeks 12 weeks 12 weeks 6 weeks	82-100%	Headache, upper respiratory tract infection, fatigue [a]. One discontinued treatment (non-treatment related)
LONESTAR, phase II trial, 2014, [38]	100 Treatment naïve, non-cirrhotic, Genotype 1	**COHORT A (n=60)** Group 1 (n=20) LDV/SOF Group 2 (n=21) LDV/SOF+RBV	8 weeks 8 weeks	95-100%	Nausea, anemia, upper respiratory tract, and headache [a]

Table 1. (Continued)

Name/Treatment group, study type/year	Patient characteristics	Treatment groups	Duration of therapy	Overall SVR rate	Adverse Events (AE)
		Group 3 (n=19) LDV/SOF	12 weeks		
		COHORT B (n=40)			
		Group 4 (n=19) SOF/LDV	12 weeks		
		Group 5 (n=21) SOF/LDV+RBV	12 weeks		
ION-1, phase III trial, 2014, [39]	865 Treatment-naïve patients Genotype 1	LDV/SOF (n=214) LDV/SOF+RBV (n=217) LDV/SOF (n=217) LDV/SOF+RBV (n=217)	12 weeks 12 weeks 24 weeks 24 weeks	97-99%	No treatment discontinuation Fatigue, headache, insomnia, nausea[a]
ION-2, phase III trial, 2014, [40]	440 treatment-experienced patients, Genotype 1	LDV/SOF (n=109) LDV/SOF+RBV (n=111) LDV/SOF (n=109) LDV/SOF+RBV (n=111)	12 weeks 12 weeks 24 weeks 24 weeks	94-99%	No treatment discontinuation Fatigue, headache, nausea[a]
ION-3, phase III clinical trial, 2014, [41]	647 treatment naïve patients without cirrhosis, Genotype 1	LDV/SOF (n=215) LDV/SOF+RBV (n=216) LDV/SOF (n=216)	8 weeks 8 weeks 12 weeks	93-95%	No treatment discontinuation, fatigue, headache, nausea, insomnia[a]
ION-4, phase III trial, 2015, [42]	335 HIV/HCV co-infected treatment-experienced patients	LDV/SOF (n=335)	12 weeks	96%	None discontinued treatment prematurely because of an AE

Name/Treatment group, study type/year	Patient characteristics	Treatment groups	Duration of therapy	Overall SVR rate	Adverse Events (AE)
Trio Health Study, Real-world study, 2016, [43]	1597 treatment naïve patients, non-cirrhotic Genotype 1	LDV/SOF±RBV (n=76) LDV/SOF (n=1521)	12 weeks 12 weeks	94-97%	Fatigue, headache, nausea [a]
HCV-TARGET observational cohort, Real-world study, 2016, [44]	2099 patients treatment-naïve, treatment-experienced, Genotype 1	(n=1788) LDV/SOF (n=282) LDV/SOF (n=910) LDV/SOF (n=510) LDV/SOF (n=86) (n=311) LDV/SOF±RBV (n=212) LDV/SOF±RBV (n=81) LDV/SOF±RBV (n=18)	8 weeks 12 weeks 24 weeks other duration 8 weeks 12 weeks other duration	>95%	13 deaths fatigue, anemia, 2 bradyarrhythmias, 1 bradycardia
SYNERGY, phase II trial, 2015, [45]	21 patients Genotype 4	LDV/SOF (n=21)	12 weeks	95%	Diarrhea, fatigue, nausea upper respiratory tract infection [a]
ASTRAL-1, phase III trial, 2015, [46]	740 patients Treatment naïve, treatment-experienced with or without cirrhosis Genotype 1, 2, 4, 5, 6	SOF/VEL (n=624) (including 35 patients from genotype 5) Placebo (n=116)	12 weeks 12 weeks	99% vs. 0%	15 patients reported serious AEs, with 1 death (cause unknown). None had serious AEs in the placebo group

Table 1. (Continued)

Name/Treatment group, study type/year	Patient characteristics	Treatment groups	Duration of therapy	Overall SVR rate	Adverse Events (AE)
ASTRAL-2, phase III trial, 2015, [47]	266 treatment naïve, treatment-experienced patients with or without cirrhosis Genotype 2	SOF/VEL (n=134) SOF+RBV (n=132)	12 weeks 12 weeks	99%	Fatigue, headache, nausea, insomnia[a]
ASTRAL-3, phase III trial, 2015, [47]	552 treatment naïve, and treatment-experienced patients with or without cirrhosis Genotype 3	SOF/VEL (n=277) SOF+RBV (n=275)	12 weeks 24 weeks	95%	Fatigue, headache, nausea, insomnia[a]
POLARIS-1, phase III trial, 2017, [20]	415 Treatment-experienced patients (with NS5A inhibitor only), Genotype 1-6	SOF/VEL/VOX (n=263) Placebo (n=152)	12 weeks 12 weeks	96% vs. 0%	Headache, fatigue, diarrhea, nausea[a]
POLARIS-2, phase III trial, 2017, [48]	941 Treatment naïve, without cirrhosis, Genotypes 1-6 (except genotype 3 and cirrhosis)	SOF/VEL/VOX (n=501) SOF/VEL (n=440)	8 weeks 12 weeks	95% vs. 98%	Headache, fatigue, diarrhea, nausea[a]
POLARIS-3, phase III trial, 2017, [48]	219 Genotype 3 with cirrhosis	SOF/VEL/VOX (n=110) SOF/VEL (n= 109)	8 weeks 12 weeks	96% for both arms	Headache, fatigue, diarrhea, nausea[a]

Name/Treatment group, study type/year	Patient characteristics	Treatment groups	Duration of therapy	Overall SVR rate	Adverse Events (AE)
POLARIS-4, phase III trial, 2017, [20]	333 Treatment-experienced (with all DAAs except NS5A inhibitors) with or without cirrhosis Genotype 1,2,3,4	SOF/VEL/VOX (n=182) SOF/VEL (n=151)	12 weeks 12 weeks	98% vs. 95%	Headache, fatigue, diarrhea, nausea[a]
SIMPLIFY, phase IV trial, 2018, [24]	103 treatment naïve or treatment-experienced patients, with recent injection drug use Genotype 1,2,3,4	SOF/VEL (n=103)	12 weeks	94%	Seven patients had a least one serious AE possibly related to therapy (rhabdomyolysis), 47% of patients had treatment-related AEs, One case of HCV reinfection was observed

Note [a] - most common adverse effect.
Abbreviations: AE, adverse event; SOF, sofosbuvir; DCV, daclatasvir; LDV, ledipasvir; VEL, velpatasvir; RBV, ribavirin; VOX, voxilaprevir; HCV, hepatitis C virus.

Table 2. Summary of AASLD-IDSA recommended Sofosbuvir-combination regimens for initial and retreatment of Hepatitis C virus Genotype 1-6

Regimen	Patient Population	Duration (weeks)	Caveats and Other Considerations
Sofosbuvir + Daclatasvir			
Genotype 1			
	Decompensated cirrhosis regardless of subtype	12	Add dose-escalating RBV[a]
	HIV/HCV coinfection when antiretroviral regimen cannot be made to accommodate recommended regimens	12	
Genotype 2			
	Decompensated cirrhosis	12	Add dose-escalating RBV[a]
	Post-liver transplant regardless of cirrhosis or decompensation	12	Add dose-escalating RBV[a]
Genotype 3			
	Decompensated cirrhosis	12	Add dose-escalating RBV[a]
	Post-liver transplant regardless of cirrhosis or decompensation	12	Add dose-escalating RBV
Genotype 4			
	Decompensated cirrhosis	12	Add dose-escalating RBV[a]
	HIV/HCV co-infection when antiretroviral regimen cannot be made to accommodate recommended regimens	12	
Ledipasvir/Sofosbuvir			
Genotype 1			
	Treatment naïve regardless of cirrhosis	12	

Regimen	Patient Population	Duration (weeks)	Caveats and Other Considerations
	Treatment naïve, no cirrhosis, non-black, HIV negative, and HCV RNA <106 IU/ml	8	
	PEG/RBV (±NS3 protease inhibitor) experienced without cirrhosis	12	
	Decompensated cirrhosis, treatment naïve or PEG/RBV (±NS3 protease inhibitor) experienced	12	Add dose-escalating RBV[a]
	Decompensated cirrhosis, prior sofosbuvir failure only	24	Add RBV
	Post-liver transplant regardless of cirrhosis or decompensation	12	Add dose-escalating RBV[a]
	Post-kidney transplant regardless of cirrhosis	12	
Genotype 4			
	Treatment naïve regardless of cirrhosis or PEG/RBV experienced without cirrhosis	12	
	Decompensated cirrhosis, treatment naïve or PEG/RBV experienced	12	Add dose-escalating RBV[a]
	Decompensated cirrhosis, sofosbuvir failure	12	Add weight-based RBV
	Post-liver transplant regardless of cirrhosis or decompensation	12	Add dose-escalating RBV[a]
	Post-kidney transplant regardless of cirrhosis	12	
Genotype 5 and 6			
	Treatment naïve or PEG/RBV experienced regardless of cirrhosis	12	
	Decompensated cirrhosis, treatment naïve or PEG/RBV experienced	12	Add dose-escalating RBV[a]
	Decompensated cirrhosis, sofosbuvir failure[b]	24	Add dose-escalating RBV[a]
	Post-liver transplant regardless of cirrhosis or decompensation	12	Add dose-escalating RBV[a]; use dose-escalating RBV if decompensated

Table 2. (Continued)

Regimen	Patient Population	Duration (weeks)	Caveats and Other Considerations
Sofosbuvir/Velpatasvir			
Genotype 1			
	Treatment naïve or PEG/RBV ± NS3 protease inhibitor-experienced regardless of cirrhosis	12	Same for GT1a and GT1b
	GT1b, non-NS5A DAA experienced regardless of cirrhosis	12	
	Decompensated cirrhosis, treatment naïve or PEG/RBV (± NS3 protease inhibitor) experienced	12	Add dose-escalating RBV[a]
	Decompensated cirrhosis, DAA failure (including NS5A)[b]	24	Add RBV
Genotype 2			
	Treatment naïve, or PEG/RBV or non-NS5A experienced regardless of cirrhosis	12	
	Decompensated cirrhosis, treatment naïve or PEG/RBV or non-NS5A experienced	12	Add weight-based RBV
	Decompensated cirrhosis, DAA failure (including sofosbuvir ± NS5A)	24	Add dose-escalating RBV
	Post-liver transplant with decompensated cirrhosis	12	Add weight-based RBV
Genotype 3			
	Treatment naïve without cirrhosis	12	
	Treatment naïve with cirrhosis or PEG/RBV experienced without cirrhosis	12	Check for Y93H RAS; if present use a different recommended regimen when available or 12 weeks of sofosbuvir/velpatasvir/voxilaprevir (an alternative regimen)[b]

Regimen	Patient Population	Duration (weeks)	Caveats and Other Considerations
	Decompensated cirrhosis, treatment naïve or PEG/RBV experienced		Add dose-escalating RBV[a]
	Decompensated cirrhosis, previously exposed to DAA (including sofosbuvir ± NS5A)[b]	24	Add weight-based RBV
	Post-liver transplant with decompensated cirrhosis	12	Add weight-based RBV
Genotype 4			
	Treatment naïve or PEG/RBV experienced regardless of cirrhosis	12	
	Decompensated cirrhosis, treatment naïve or PEG/RBV (± NS3 protease inhibitor) experienced	12	Add weight-based RBV[a]
	Decompensated cirrhosis, DAA failure (including NS5A)[b]	24	Add weight-based RBV
Genotype 5 and 6			
	Treatment naïve or PEG/RBV experienced regardless of cirrhosis	12	
	Decompensated cirrhosis, treatment naïve or PEG/RBV (±NS3 protease inhibitor) experienced	12	Add weight-based RBV (extend treatment to 24 weeks if RBV ineligible)
	Decompensated cirrhosis, DAA failure (including NS5A)[b]	24	Add weight-based RBV
Sofosbuvir/Velpatasvir/Voxilaprevir			
Genotype 1			
	NS5A failure (including NS3 protease inhibitor) regardless of cirrhosis	12	Same for GT1a and GT1b
	GT1a, non-NS5A failures (including NS3 protease inhibitors) regardless of cirrhosis	12	
	Not for decompensated cirrhosis or post-liver transplant with cirrhosis		

Table 2. (Continued)

Regimen	Patient Population	Duration (weeks)	Caveats and Other Considerations
Genotype 2			
	NS5A failures	12	
	Not for decompensated cirrhosis or post-liver transplant with cirrhosis		
Genotype 3			
	PEG/RBV experienced with cirrhosis, or DAA failure (including NS5A inhibitors) regardless of cirrhosis	12	Add RBV for prior NS5A inhibitor failure and cirrhosis
	Not for decompensated cirrhosis or post-liver transplant with cirrhosis		
Genotype 4, 5, 6			
	NS5A failures (including NS3 protease inhibitors) regardless of cirrhosis	12	
	Not for decompensated cirrhosis or post-liver transplant with cirrhosis		
Sofosbuvir + Elbasvir/Grazoprevir			
Genotype 3			
	PEG/RBV experienced with compensated cirrhosis	12	
	Not for decompensated cirrhosis or post-liver transplant with cirrhosis		

Source: Panel, A.-I.H.G., Hepatitis C Guidance 2018 Update: AASLD-IDSA Recommendations for Testing, Managing, and Treating Hepatitis C Virus Infection. Clin Infect Dis, 2018. **67**(10): p. 1477-1492.

Note: [a] extend treatment to 24 weeks if RBV ineligible, [b] off-label use.

In the early access "Autorisation Temporaire d'Utilisation" program, real-world data supported the effectiveness of the DCV+SOF combination with or without RBV in HCV/HIV co-infected patients with advanced liver disease. Six hundred seventeen patients were assessed for safety, and 407 patients were assessed for efficacy. The population included mostly patients with hepatic cirrhosis (72% of whom 18% were decompensated), HCV GT 1 (69%), 3 (12%), 4 (19%) and HCV treatment-experienced (82%). Overall modified intention-to-treat SVR12 was 92% (95% without cirrhosis; 90% with cirrhosis). SVR12 was found to be consistent among GTs 1, 3 and 4, and other combined antiretroviral regimens. Safety analysis of the 617 patients yielded 7 who discontinued treatment and 10 on- or off-treatment deaths, 3 of the patients who discontinued treatment were reported to be subsequently fatal (hepatic carcinoma, decompensated cirrhosis/multi-organ failure, respiratory distress). Three non-fatal discontinuations were due to treatment-related lymphopenia, renal insufficiency, and attempted suicide, and 1 non-treatment related due to anxiety/ascites/hepatocellular carcinoma/pneumonia/ encephalopathy. The investigators concluded that the combination of DCV and SOF with or without RBV was well tolerated in the real-world populations of HIC/HCV co-infected individuals with advanced liver disease. Limitations to this study were that current or former PWID receiving opioid substitutions and IDU were not captured, although they noted the likelihood that many patients in this real-world study would have been part of this cohort [36].

Recently, there have been few data on the efficacy and safety of DCV and SOF regimens for people with mental illness. In a recent prospective observational study, 17 patients receiving DAA treatments, SOF + DCV combination (n=7/17), SOF + Simeprevir (SMV) (n=9/17) and LDV/SOF (n=1/17) were followed and assessed for adherence, treatment response and psychiatric symptoms [21]. In this study, it was noted that DAA treatment did not increase depressive symptoms or influence sleep quality in any way. It was noted that the Beck Depression Inventory (BDI) scores decreased after SOF treatment, suggesting an improvement in mental health parameters. Moreover, it was noted that adherence to treatment was consistent high (>95%) as well as treatment response (88%), although the sample size of this study limits its generalizability [21].

2.2. Efficacy and Safety of Sofosbuvir and Ledipasvir Combination

The once a day Ledipasvir (LDV)/SOF fixed-dose combination with or without RBV has been evaluated extensively in pivotal studies, including LONESTAR, ELECTRON-2, ION-1, ION-2, ION-3, and 4 [37-42]. In the ION studies, genotype 1 was evaluated using LDV/SOF or LDV/SOF with RBV and was found to have consistently high rates of SVR12 across all arms (Table 1). ION-1 assessed treatment-naïve patients with and without cirrhosis, ION-2 looked at interferon-experienced patients with and without cirrhosis and ION-3 evaluated treatment –naïve patients without cirrhosis. Presence of baseline NS5A resistance-associated variants (RAV) among treatment-naïve non-cirrhotic patients in the ION-1 trial had slightly lower SVR12 rates when compared to those without RAVs (96% vs. 99% respectively) [39]. There were no treatment-related discontinuations, and the most common adverse effects were fatigue, headache, and nausea. Of note, patients who had RBV included in the regimen had higher rates of fatigue, insomnia, asthenia, rash, cough, pruritus, and anemia (all known to be RBV-associated adverse effects) when compared to the groups that received RBV [39-42]. Currently, the LDV/SOF combination is indicated for HCV GT 1 treatment naïve patients with or without compensated cirrhosis for 12 weeks, with a shorter treatment duration for those who are non-black, HIV-negative non-cirrhotic patients whose HCV RNA is <6million IU/mL [31, 49]. In the SYNERGY study conducted by Kohli et al. the use of this combination was also assessed for 21 patients with GT4, 60% of which was treatment naïve, and 43% had advanced cirrhosis. Overall SVR rate after 12 weeks was 95% and was well tolerated by the patients with no patients discontinuing treatment [45].

Other small studies supported the use of LDV/SOF combinations for GTs 5 and 6, although data is limited at best [50-52]. In a study conducted by Abergel et al., a phase 2 trial was done at five hospitals in France where 41 patients with GT5 were recruited; 21 who are treatment naïve and 20 who were treatment-experienced. Thirty-nine out of 41 achieved SVR12 overall. The most common AEs were asthenia (39%), headache (27%), and fatigue (10%) [50]. In another phase 2 study, Gane et al. evaluated 126 patients with GT 3 and 6 using LDV/SOF with or without RBV. Fifty-one patients were treatment naïve with HCV GT3, and 50 were treatment-experienced. Twenty-five patients were treatment naïve, or treatment-experienced and had GT6. SVR12 for HCV GT6 was 96%, while GT3 patients had 100% and 82% for treatment naïve and treatment-experienced respectively. The most common AEs were a headache, upper respiratory tract infection, and fatigue [52].

Efficacies of these trials are consistently reflected in large real-world studies for the 8-week and 12-week courses for treatment naïve patients who are non-cirrhotic with HCV GT1 (HCV-TARGET, TRIO study) [43, 44].

To assess the safety and efficacy of LDV/SOF among PWID, Grebely et al., evaluated patients receiving OST with buprenorphine or methadone and drug use using data from phase 3 ION studies. Among the 1952 patients enrolled, 4% (n=70) were receiving OST. The study found that there was no difference in treatment completion (97% vs. 98%, p= 0.40), ≥80% adherence (93% vs. 92%, p =1.00), SVR12 (94% vs. 97%, *p*=0.28) and serious adverse effects (4% vs. 3%; *p=0.43*) when comparing OST vs. non-OST. The researchers concluded that the use of LDV/SOF is safe and effective among PWID receiving OST and those with illicit drug use during HCV therapy, although its generalizability is limited due to its small sample size and exclusion of active drug use.

The real-world study of Gayam et al. also evaluated the efficacy and safety of LDV/SOF ± RBV combination among patients who abuse drugs and those who are on OST. One hundred eighty-one patients on LDV/SOF ± RBV were retrospectively analyzed, and results yielded 90.1% (n=163/181) SVR rate after 12 weeks post-treatment for both groups [53].

On subgroup analysis of PWUD, it was found that 94 out of 101 (93.1%) of patients on this regimen achieved SVR 12, which mirrors previously done clinical and real-world studies.

On the other hand, Tang et al. evaluated SOF/LDV regimens in people with mental illness with the ERADICATE and SYNERGY-A trials [54]. It was found that 100% of SVR12 rates were achieved by both studies (ERADICATE, n=7/7, SYNERGY n=15/15) and yielded no statistical difference when compared to those without mental illness. Furthermore, there were high treatment adherence rates in both trials ranging from 97% - 98%. Mean BDI scores also decreased from 5.24 at baseline to 3.28 during treatment and 2.82 post-treatment, suggesting an improvement of mental illness with the use of SOF-based therapies. The investigators concluded that the use of SOF-based therapies is effective, and is a viable treatment option for people with mental illness, dispelling the notion of lower adherence to treatment in patients with mental illness [54].

2.3. Efficacy and Safety of Sofosbuvir and Velpatasvir Combination

The advent of the fixed-dose combination of SOF and the NS5A inhibitor Velpatasvir (VEL) has paved the way for a simpler treatment regimen for those infected with CHC. It is approved by the FDA for all HCV GTs to treat adult patients with CHC with or without compensated cirrhosis. Efficacy and safety of this regimen were evaluated by the ASTRAL and POLARIS-2, POLARIS-3, and POLARIS-4 trials (Table 1). In ASTRAL-1, overall SVR12 rate for 624 treatment naïve or treatment-experienced patients (with an NS3 protease inhibitor) with GT 1,2,4,5,6 was 97-99% as compared to 0% with placebo. This result did not change regardless of cirrhosis status (n=120/121, 99% for cirrhotic patients) and baseline NS5A RAVs [46]. SVR12 was also high (n=48/48, 100%) for those who had prior treatment failure with a protease inhibitor plus peg-IFN/RBV [46]. POLARIS-2 corroborated this result by randomizing 941 patients to 8 weeks of SOF/VEL/Voxilaprevir (VOX) or 12 weeks of

SOF/VEL, which yielded consistently high SVR12 rates for all GTs with or without cirrhosis (99% vs. 97% respectively) [48]. In ASTRAL-2 662 patients given SOF/VEL remained superior compared to SOF+RBV with an overall SVR12 rate of 99% vs. 95% respectively, for patients with HCV GT2 infection [47]. For those with GT3, ASTRAL-3 demonstrated the superiority of SOF/VEL for 12 weeks vs. 24 weeks of SOF plus RBV for both treatments naïve or treatment-experienced patients (95% vs. 80% respectively). SVR12 rate for patients with compensated cirrhosis in this study was 93% (n=40/43) [47]. The most usual AEs reported for the ASTRAL trials were fatigue, headache, nausea, and insomnia [46, 47]. Mostly, serious AEs were reported in 15 patients in the SOF/VEL group of ASTRAL-1, including 1 death from unknown causes. None had an AE with the placebo group [46]. Lastly, POLARIS-4 also evaluated 12 weeks of SOF/VEL in non-NS5A inhibitor-DAA experienced patients and was found to have high SVR12 rates for both HCV GT1b and 2 (95% and 97% respectively), suggesting a good alternative option to SOF/VEL/VOX within these populations [20].

In one study, Grebely, et al. did a post hoc analysis of the efficacy, safety, and tolerability of SOF/VEL among the participants of OST within the ASTRAL trials. Of the 1035 patients enrolled, (ASTRAL1, (n=624); ASTRAL-2, (n=134) and ASTRAL-3, (n=277)), patients were stratified by receipt of OST 51 (5%) at enrollment (67% methadone, 33% buprenorphine) vs. those with No OST (n=984). The overall SVR12 rate was 96% between those receiving OST when compared to those not receiving OST (98%). Adherence to ≥90% of therapy was 90% among OST participants, and completion of therapy was at 96%. AEs were mostly mild to moderate severity, while serious AEs in those receiving OST included abdominal pain (n=1), bronchitis (n=1) and palpitation (n=1). The study concluded that the SOF/VEL combination was well tolerated and effective among people receiving OST [55]. The small sample size of this study and the exclusion of recent IDU limited it to be generalizable to other PWID populations. The SIMPLIFY trial addressed these limitations, where recent IDU (within the past 6 months) were evaluated to address the gap in knowledge regarding the treatment of PWID in patients having

CHC (Table 1). In this phase 4 trial, 103 patients with GT 1-4 was given the SOF/VEL combination once daily for 12 weeks. Overall SVR12 of the cohort was 94%, which included two failures due to lost to follow-up and one that died due to an overdose. Only one serious AE was observed (rhabdomyolysis), which was possibly related to therapy. The researchers concluded that IDU before or during treatment did not affect SVR12 and that HCV treatment should be encouraged to all patients irrespective of drug use [24].

There is scarce data available specifically on the treatment response of SOF/VEL among patients with mental illness. Although one recent study included this regimen, where they analyzed 48 veterans receiving DAA treatment. Fourteen of the 48 patients received SOF/VEL, while the others had elbasvir/grazoprevir (n=30/48) or SOF/LDV 4(n=4/48). Patient Health Questionnaires (PHQ-9) were analyzed, showing decreasing trends from baseline to end-of-treatment for all subjects except for the SOF/VEL group, although there was no statistical significance observed [56]. This implies that DAA regimens do not have mood decompensations during treatment and can be safely used, as compared to previous IFN-based therapies.

2.4. Efficacy and Safety Sofosbuvir/Velpatasvir/Voxilaprevir Combination

In 2017, retreatment options for adult patients with CHC with or without cirrhosis had expanded with the FDA approval of the fixed-dose combination of SOF/VEL and VOX, an NS3/4A inhibitor. Previously, the addition of RBV or longer treatment durations were used to retreat persons who received prior DAA treatment. Currently, SOF/VEL/VOX is indicated for all HCV GTs who have been previously treated with an HCV regimen containing an NS5A inhibitor, or for GT 1a or 3 infections and have been previously treated with an HCV regimen containing SOF without an NS5A inhibitor [57]. POLARIS-1 and POLARIS-4 evaluated treatment-experienced patients with DAA containing regimens (with NS5A inhibitors only), and DAA containing regimens (except NS5A inhibitors) with or without cirrhosis respectively (Table 1). In POLARIS-1, overall SVR12 rate of SOF/VEL/VOX compared to placebo was high (96%), while those patients with and without cirrhosis had SVR12 rates of 93% vs. 99% respectively [20]. In POLARIS-4, overall SVR12 rate of SOF/VEL/VOX was 98%, while the SOF/VEL combination was 90%. Although the study was not powered for a comparison between these two regimens, superiority was achieved only for the SOF/VEL/VOX group vs. SOF/VEL group based on a designed performance goal of 85% (p<0.001 vs. p=0.09 respectively) [20]. The most common AEs observed for both POLARIS-1 and POLARIS-4 was a headache, fatigue, diarrhea, and nausea; no patients discontinued treatment due to the events [20].

Recently, a real-world trial assessed the effectiveness in 573 DAA-experienced was done by Belperio et al., at 104 Veteran's affairs facilities and was given 12 weeks of SOF/VEL/VOX combination in clinical practice. Overall SVR12 rates for GT1 was 90.7% (n=429/473), GT2 90% (n=18/20), GT3 91.3% (n=42/46) and GT4 100% (n=12). The population consisted of mostly male (99%) with an overall cohort of 63.6 years old. Of note, patients with GT1, GT2, and GT3 had lower SVR12 rates when SOF/VEL was used before treatment with SOF/VEL/VOX (78.9%, 86.7%, and 84.6% respectively). Although this is the largest real-world study to date, the generalizability of GT2 and GT4 is limited due to the small sample size [58].

No trials have been done for SOF/VEL/VOX in patients with mental illness or those who use drugs to date. Research on this population may be warranted in future studies to address the need of these vulnerable populations.

3. SCREENING OF HEPATITIS C INFECTED PERSONS IN PEOPLE WITH MENTAL ILLNESS AND SUBSTANCE USE DISORDERS

As mentioned earlier, there is an increased emphasis on screening HCV among persons with substance use disorders and mental illness due to the high comorbidity of these diseases. Almost half of these high-risk populations for HCV remain undiagnosed; most persons afflicted with HCV are not aware of their disease; they only seek medical care when they develop liver-related complications [59, 60]. To reduce the burden of HCV disease overall, selective screening has been advocated by numerous health organizations for people at risk for HCV infection (e.g., SMI and people with substance use disorders). [2, 5, 31], Screening involves measurement of antibody to HCV which is highly sensitive and specific, although a positive result requires confirmation by nucleic acid testing for the detection of HCV RNA for persons who are chronically infected [2, 61].

Currently, the Centers for Disease Control (CDC) and United States Prevention Services Task Force (USPTSF) recommend screening for Hepatitis C among all individuals born in 1945-1965, and that high-risk populations be screened as well [62]. The AASLD-IDSA also recommend annual HCV testing for PWID with no prior testing or past negative testing and subsequent IDU. Depending on the level of risk, more frequent testing may be indicated [31]. Lastly, screening for illicit drug use should also be done for persons seeking services for infectious diseases (e.g., HIV, STDs, viral hepatitis, and TB), due to its high prevalence within this population. By adequately identifying these high-risk individuals, proper counseling can be initiated, and referral to relevant prevention and treatment programs can be started, leading to safer behaviors and overall risk reduction and eventual decrease in the burden of the disease [5].

4. LINKAGE TO CARE AND INTEGRATION OF SERVICES FOR HCV-INFECTED PSYCHIATRIC PATIENTS AND PERSONS WHO USE DRUGS

Ensuring proper linkage to effective treatment is crucial to reduce the prevalence of HCV infection at all levels. This is especially crucial for at-risk populations, including PWUD and/or have co-occurring mental illness [63]. For example, in their review of 13 studies from North America,

Hughes and colleagues found approximately 1 in 5 patients with SMI was infected with the HCV [6]. This finding is in keeping with a 2011 comprehensive review of the prevalence of physical illnesses among individuals with SMI [64]. The authors found a reported 19.6% of persons with SMI have HCV infection and that its transmission correlated highly with participants' pattern of drug use and sexual behavior.

Similarly, Himelhoch et al.'s study of United States' veterans found the odds of being diagnosed with HCV in persons with co-occurring substance use disorder and schizophrenia or bipolar disorder is approximately 6 to 7 times the odds of HCV in similar patients but who don't have a history of substance use disorder [65]. In a separate review of over 113,900 individuals with HCV who presented to US Veterans Affairs facilities between 1999 and 2003, only approximately 12 percent received treatment [66]. Additionally, the authors found, among other factors, that psychiatric and substance use disorders, including schizophrenia, bipolar disorder, and alcohol abuse, correlated positively with HCV non-treatment [66].

Despite the high burden of disease, a disproportionate number of HCV patients who have co-occurring mental and/or substance use disorders face significant barriers to treatment [63]. Knowledge of factors impacting treatment of HCV patients is crucial to developing treatment strategies. Few evidence-based, public health/clinical strategies have been established to address the disparity in healthcare and the resulting higher prevalence of HCV infection among vulnerable populations including those with SMI [31, 67]. It is worth noting that a comprehensive healthcare delivery approach that integrates clinical care (e.g., coordination of the expertise of a nurse, internist, psychiatrist, social worker etc.) and public health (e.g., patient education and counseling, case management etc.) is more effective than stand-alone health delivery models in the management of patients with dual diagnosis and co-morbid HCV infection.

The seminal work of Rosenberg and colleagues in 2004 describes a brief "*screen, test, immunize, reduce risk, and refer* (STIRR)" intervention that brings "a small group of expert providers to a clinical site, for a limited period, to provide core services to an undertreated, at-risk population"; this can be likened to the mobile crisis units that offer around the clock services to psychiatric patients in the community. The STIRR approach ultimately reduces/eliminates the barrier to the management of HCV and HIV among patients with mental illness and substance use disorder [67]. While the STIRR methodology has already been published, and questions regarding the intervention can be addressed to the lead author, a brief description of its core components is as follows:

1) Establishing the intervention team consisting of, but not limited to, an internist with expertise in diagnosis and treatment of viral hepatitis and HIV, a psychiatrist versed in the management of patients with dual diagnosis, a nurse, and administrative personnel. Additionally, the team ensures that the resources required to support their smooth operation (e.g., materials for laboratory testing and storage of hepatitis vaccine) and referral of patients for additional services are in place.
2) Seeking organizational support for the intervention's implementation at target healthcare sites by meeting with key stakeholders to introduce the STIRR model. Among other issues, the burden of infectious disease in the population, as well as the resources required and barriers to implementation, are determined.
3) Provision of on-site services, which elaborates on the wide range of services offered by the STIRR nurse to patients at three different points of contact. These include in-depth, pretest education and counseling about viral hepatitis and HIV, risk assessment, blood testing, and immunization with the combination vaccine, Twinrix, which offers protection against both Hepatitis A and hepatitis B. Of note, there is currently no vaccine against HCV; hence, the focus of intervention is to identify early and treat those infected with the virus.
4) Referring patients for further management and providing technical support to other health providers.

A dynamic, evidence-based, guidance document on HCV management have also been published by the AASLD-IDSA [31]. The document, however, is targeted to U.S. clinicians and includes recommendations on screening and management of HCV-infected persons. Although, the AASLD-IDSA did not specifically mention patients with mental illness, their recommendations regarding PWID are relevant because a disproportionate number of PWUD have mental illness [68]. For example, it is highly recommended that "PWID should be offered linkage to *harm reduction services* when available, including needle/syringe service programs and substance use disorder treatment programs."

As mentioned earlier, AASLD-IDSA also recommends that the management of patients with HCV infection be multidisciplinary. This is crucial to not only treat HCV infection but also to address co-occurring disorders (e.g., psychiatric and substance use disorders) that significantly increase the risk for HCV re-infection. Because PWID is often the subject of discrimination by healthcare professionals due to countertransferential reactions, they may receive less adequate treatment [69, 70]. Therefore, healthcare providers should be conscious of this inherent bias and are encouraged to offer proper treatment of HCV regardless of drug-use status. Furthermore, current recommendations are to offer HCV treatment alongside syringe exchange programs and medication-assisted treatment (e.g., opioid treatment programs). Other novel approaches that are recommended include using case managers to help facilitate coordination of care with treatment facilities and establishing programs that offer free HCV screening and treatment [71-73].

In keeping with the recommendations of AASLD-IDSA and other health organizations, analysis of integrated models of care has seen success in removing barriers to treatment of HCV [72, 74]. In a study by Harris et al., the establishment of a program of comprehensive on-site hepatitis C care in one Methadone Maintenance Treatment Program (MMTP) composed of an Internist, Psychiatrist, Physician's assistant, nursing and substance abuse staff was trained to coordinate their services and offer comprehensive support to their patients. Their study highlighted that by integrating all services in one area, patients had access to a broader range of services which translated to in an increase in identification of HCV infected individuals, adherence to treatment and therefore, a decrease in the total burden of the disease [74].

CONCLUSION

SOF-based IFN-free combinations have changed the way treatment is delivered to people with mental illness and substance use disorders. Excellent safety profiles, high SVR12 rates and simplicity of use have paved the way for the goal reduction of overall HCV burden, and the eventual eradication of HCV infection. Further studies need to be undertaken to address concerns of treatment adherence and response among these high-risk populations, although integration of services and linkage to care is arguably a step forward in the right direction in tackling these concerns.

REFERENCES

[1] Petruzziello, A., et al., Global epidemiology of hepatitis C virus infection: An up-date of the distribution and circulation of hepatitis C virus genotypes. *World J Gastroenterol,* 2016. 22(34): p. 7824-40.

[2] WHO, Guidelines for the screening, care and treatment of persons with hepatitis C infection Updated version, April 2016. 2016: France.

[3] Brown, C. R., J. H. MacLachlan, and B. C. Cowie, Addressing the increasing global burden of viral hepatitis. *Hepatobiliary Surg Nutr,* 2017. 6(4): p. 274-276.

[4] Philip Aston, K. C., Haley O'Farrell, Alex Cassenote, Cassia J. Mendes-Correa, Aluisio Segurado, Phuong Hoang, George Lankford and Hien Tran, Hepatitis C Viral Dynamics Using a Combination Therapy of Interferon, Ribavirin, and Telaprevir: Mathematical Modeling and Model Validation, I. Shahid, Editor. 2018, Intechopen.

[5] Centers for Disease, C. and Prevention, Integrated prevention services for HIV infection, viral hepatitis, sexually transmitted diseases, and tuberculosis for persons who use drugs illicitly: summary guidance from CDC and the U.S. Department of Health and Human Services. *MMWR Recomm Rep,* 2012. 61(RR-5): p. 1-40.

[6] Hughes, E., et al., Prevalence of HIV, hepatitis B, and hepatitis C in people with severe mental illness: a systematic review and meta-analysis. *Lancet Psychiatry,* 2016. 3(1): p. 40-48.

[7] Nelson, P. K., et al., Global epidemiology of hepatitis B and hepatitis C in people who inject drugs: results of systematic reviews. *Lancet,* 2011. 378(9791): p. 571-83.

[8] Omland, L. H., et al., Socioeconomic status in HCV infected patients - risk and prognosis. *Clin Epidemiol,* 2013. 5: p. 163-72.

[9] Trager, E., et al., Hepatitis C Screening Rate Among Underserved Adults With Serious Mental Illness Receiving Care in California Community Mental Health Centers. *Am J Public Health,* 2016. 106(4): p. 740-2.

[10] Friedland, G., Infectious disease comorbidities adversely affecting substance users with HIV: hepatitis C and tuberculosis. *J Acquir Immune Defic Syndr,* 2010. 55 Suppl 1: p. S37-42.

[11] Dinwiddie, S. H., L. Shicker, and T. Newman, Prevalence of hepatitis C among psychiatric patients in the public sector. *Am J Psychiatry,* 2003. 160(1): p. 172-4.

[12] Manns, M. P., H. Wedemeyer, and M. Cornberg, Treating viral hepatitis C: efficacy, side effects, and complications. *Gut,* 2006. 55(9): p. 1350-9.

[13] Fried, M. W., Side effects of therapy of hepatitis C and their management. *Hepatology,* 2002. 36(5 Suppl 1): p. S237-44.

[14] Palumbo, E., Pegylated interferon and ribavirin treatment for hepatitis C virus infection. *Ther Adv Chronic Dis,* 2011. 2(1): p. 39-45.

[15] Butt, A. A. and F. Kanwal, Boceprevir and telaprevir in the management of hepatitis C virus-infected patients. *Clin Infect Dis,* 2012. 54(1): p. 96-104.

[16] Hezode, C., et al., Triple therapy in treatment-experienced patients with HCV-cirrhosis in a multicentre cohort of the French Early Access Programme (ANRS CO20-CUPIC) - NCT01514890. *J Hepatol,* 2013. 59(3): p. 434-41.

[17] Yu, M. L., Hepatitis C treatment from "response-guided" to "resource-guided" therapy in the transition era from interferon-containing to interferon-free regimens. *J Gastroenterol Hepatol,* 2017. 32(8): p. 1436-1442.

[18] Li, G. and E. De Clercq, Current therapy for chronic hepatitis C: The role of direct-acting antivirals. *Antiviral Res,* 2017. 142: p. 83-122.

[19] Chopra, D. and B. Bhandari, Sofosbuvir: really meets the unmet needs for Hepatis C treatment ? *Infect Disord Drug Targets,* 2018.

[20] Bourliere, M., et al., Sofosbuvir, Velpatasvir, and Voxilaprevir for Previously Treated HCV Infection. *N Engl J Med,* 2017. 376(22): p. 2134-2146.

[21] Sundberg, I., et al., Direct-acting antiviral treatment in real world patients with hepatitis C not associated with psychiatric side effects: a prospective observational study. *BMC Psychiatry,* 2018. 18(1): p. 157.

[22] Alimohammadi, A., et al., Real-world Efficacy of Direct-Acting Antiviral Therapy for HCV Infection Affecting People Who Inject Drugs Delivered in a Multidisciplinary Setting. *Open Forum Infect Dis,* 2018. 5(6): p. ofy120.

[23] Grebely, J., et al., Sofosbuvir-Based Direct-Acting Antiviral Therapies for HCV in People Receiving Opioid Substitution Therapy: An Analysis of Phase 3 Studies. *Open Forum Infect Dis,* 2018. 5(2): p. ofy001.

[24] Grebely, J., et al., Sofosbuvir and velpatasvir for hepatitis C virus infection in people with recent injection drug use (SIMPLIFY): an open-label, single-arm, phase 4, multicentre trial. *Lancet Gastroenterol Hepatol,* 2018. 3(3): p. 153-161.

[25] Gallach, M., et al., Impact of treatment with direct-acting antivirals on anxiety and depression in chronic hepatitis C. *PLOS ONE,* 2018. 13(12): p. e0208112.

[26] Collins, L. F., et al., Direct-Acting Antivirals Improve Access to Care and Cure for Patients With HIV and Chronic HCV Infection. *Open Forum Infect Dis,* 2018. 5(1): p. ofx264.
[27] Jain, M. K., et al., Has Access to Hepatitis C Virus Therapy Changed for Patients With Mental Health or Substance Use Disorders in the Direct-Acting-Antiviral Period? *Hepatology,* 2019. 69(1): p. 51-63.
[28] Socias, M. E., et al., Disparities in uptake of direct-acting antiviral therapy for hepatitis C among people who inject drugs in a Canadian setting. *Liver Int,* 2019.
[29] Grebely, J., et al., Elimination of HCV as a public health concern among people who inject drugs by 2030 - What will it take to get there? *J Int AIDS Soc,* 2017. 20(1): p. 22146.
[30] Barua, S., et al., Restrictions for Medicaid Reimbursement of Sofosbuvir for the Treatment of Hepatitis C Virus Infection in the United States. *Ann Intern Med,* 2015. 163(3): p. 215-23.
[31] Panel, A. I. H. G., Hepatitis C Guidance 2018 Update: AASLD-IDSA Recommendations for Testing, Managing, and Treating Hepatitis C Virus Infection. *Clin Infect Dis,* 2018. 67(10): p. 1477-1492.
[32] Sulkowski, M. S., et al., Daclatasvir plus sofosbuvir for previously treated or untreated chronic HCV infection. *N Engl J Med*, 2014. 370(3): p. 211-21.
[33] Poordad, F., et al., Daclatasvir with sofosbuvir and ribavirin for hepatitis C virus infection with advanced cirrhosis or post-liver transplantation recurrence. *Hepatology,* 2016. 63(5): p. 1493-505.
[34] Wyles, D. L., et al., Daclatasvir plus Sofosbuvir for HCV in Patients Coinfected with HIV-1. *N Engl J Med*, 2015. 373(8): p. 714-25.
[35] Nelson, D. R., et al., All-oral 12-week treatment with daclatasvir plus sofosbuvir in patients with hepatitis C virus genotype 3 infection: ALLY-3 phase III study. *Hepatology,* 2015. 61(4): p. 1127-35.
[36] Lacombe, K., et al., Real-World Efficacy of Daclatasvir and Sofosbuvir, With and Without Ribavirin, in HIV/HCV Coinfected Patients With Advanced Liver Disease in a French Early Access Cohort. *J Acquir Immune Defic Syndr,* 2017. 75(1): p. 97-107.

[37] Gane, E. J., et al., Efficacy of nucleotide polymerase inhibitor sofosbuvir plus the NS5A inhibitor ledipasvir or the NS5B non-nucleoside inhibitor GS-9669 against HCV genotype 1 infection. *Gastroenterology,* 2014. 146(3): p. 736-743 e1.
[38] Lawitz, E., et al., Sofosbuvir and ledipasvir fixed-dose combination with and without ribavirin in treatment-naive and previously treated patients with genotype 1 hepatitis C virus infection (LONESTAR): an open-label, randomised, phase 2 trial. *Lancet,* 2014. 383(9916): p. 515-23.
[39] Afdhal, N., et al., Ledipasvir and sofosbuvir for untreated HCV genotype 1 infection. *N Engl J Med,* 2014. 370(20): p. 1889-98.
[40] Afdhal, N., et al., Ledipasvir and sofosbuvir for previously treated HCV genotype 1 infection. *N Engl J Med,* 2014. 370(16): p. 1483-93.
[41] Kowdley, K. V., et al., Ledipasvir and sofosbuvir for 8 or 12 weeks for chronic HCV without cirrhosis. *N Engl J Med,* 2014. 370(20): p. 1879-88.
[42] Naggie, S., et al., Ledipasvir and Sofosbuvir for HCV in Patients Coinfected with HIV-1. *N Engl J Med,* 2015. 373(8): p. 705-13.
[43] Tapper, E. B., et al., Real-world effectiveness for 12 weeks of ledipasvir-sofosbuvir for genotype 1 hepatitis C: the Trio Health study. *J Viral Hepat,* 2017. 24(1): p. 22-27.
[44] Terrault, N. A., et al., Effectiveness of Ledipasvir-Sofosbuvir Combination in Patients With Hepatitis C Virus Infection and Factors Associated With Sustained Virologic Response. *Gastroenterology,* 2016. 151(6): p. 1131-1140 e5.
[45] Kohli, A., et al., Ledipasvir and sofosbuvir for hepatitis C genotype 4: a proof-of-concept, single-centre, open-label phase 2a cohort study. *Lancet Infect Dis,* 2015. 15(9): p. 1049-1054.
[46] Feld, J. J., et al., Sofosbuvir and Velpatasvir for HCV Genotype 1, 2, 4, 5, and 6 Infection. *N Engl J Med,* 2015. 373(27): p. 2599-607.
[47] Foster, G. R., et al., Sofosbuvir and Velpatasvir for HCV Genotype 2 and 3 Infection. *N Engl J Med,* 2015. 373(27): p. 2608-17.
[48] Jacobson, I. M., et al., Efficacy of 8 Weeks of Sofosbuvir, Velpatasvir, and Voxilaprevir in Patients With Chronic HCV

Infection: 2 Phase 3 Randomized Trials. *Gastroenterology,* 2017. 153(1): p. 113-122.
[49] Inc., G. S. *HARVONI US full Prescribing Information.* November 2017; Available from: https://www.gilead.com/~/media/Files/pdfs/medicines/liver-disease/harvoni/harvoni_pi.pdf.
[50] Abergel, A., et al., Ledipasvir-sofosbuvir in patients with hepatitis C virus genotype 5 infection: an open-label, multicentre, single-arm, phase 2 study. *Lancet Infect Dis,* 2016. 16(4): p. 459-64.
[51] Nguyen, M. H., et al., Open Label Study of 8 vs. 12 Weeks of Ledipasvir/Sofosbuvir in Genotype 6 Treatment Naive or Experienced Patients. *Am J Gastroenterol,* 2017. 112(12): p. 1824-1831.
[52] Gane, E. J., et al., Efficacy of ledipasvir and sofosbuvir, with or without ribavirin, for 12 weeks in patients with HCV genotype 3 or 6 infection. *Gastroenterology,* 2015. 149(6): p. 1454-1461 e1.
[53] Gayam, V., et al., Real-world study of hepatitis C treatment with direct-acting antivirals in patients with drug abuse and opioid agonist therapy. *Scand J Gastroenterol,* 2019. 54(5): p. 646-655.
[54] Tang, L. S., et al., Safe and effective sofosbuvir-based therapy in patients with mental health disease on hepatitis C virus treatment. *World J Hepatol,* 2016. 8(31): p. 1318-1326.
[55] Grebely, J., et al., Efficacy and Safety of Sofosbuvir/Velpatasvir in Patients With Chronic Hepatitis C Virus Infection Receiving Opioid Substitution Therapy: Analysis of Phase 3 ASTRAL Trials. *Clin Infect Dis,* 2016. 63(11): p. 1479-1481.
[56] Sackey, B., et al., Evaluating psychiatric outcomes associated with direct-acting antiviral treatment in veterans with hepatitis C infection. *Mental Health Clinician,* 2018. 8(3): p. 116-121.
[57] Gilead Sciences, I. VOSEVI full Prescribing Information. November 2017.
[58] Belperio, P. S., et al., Real-world effectiveness of sofosbuvir/velpatasvir/voxilaprevir in 573 direct-acting antiviral experienced hepatitis C patients. *J Viral Hepat,* 2019.

[59] Zuure, F. R., et al., Outcomes of hepatitis C screening programs targeted at risk groups hidden in the general population: a systematic review. *BMC Public Health*, 2014. 14: p. 66.
[60] Denniston, M. M., et al., Awareness of infection, knowledge of hepatitis C, and medical follow-up among individuals testing positive for hepatitis C: National Health and Nutrition Examination Survey 2001-2008. *Hepatology*, 2012. 55(6): p. 1652-61.
[61] Chevaliez, S. and J. M. Pawlotsky, Hepatitis C virus serologic and virologic tests and clinical diagnosis of HCV-related liver disease. *Int J Med Sci*, 2006. 3(2): p. 35-40.
[62] Moyer, V. A. and U. S. P. S. T. Force, Screening for hepatitis C virus infection in adults: U.S. Preventive Services Task Force recommendation statement. *Ann Intern Med*, 2013. 159(5): p. 349-57.
[63] Ho, S. B., et al., Integrated Care Increases Treatment and Improves Outcomes of Patients With Chronic Hepatitis C Virus Infection and Psychiatric Illness or Substance Abuse. *Clin Gastroenterol Hepatol*, 2015. 13(11): p. 2005-14 e1-3.
[64] M, D. E. H., et al., Physical illness in patients with severe mental disorders. I. Prevalence, impact of medications and disparities in health care. *World Psychiatry*, 2011. 10(1): p. 52-77.
[65] Himelhoch, S., et al., Understanding associations between serious mental illness and hepatitis C virus among veterans: a national multivariate analysis. *Psychosomatics*, 2009. 50(1): p. 30-7.
[66] Edlin, B. R., Hepatitis C screening: getting it right. *Hepatology*, 2013. 57(4): p. 1644-50.
[67] Rosenberg, S., et al., The STIRR model of best practices for blood-borne diseases among clients with serious mental illness. *Psychiatr Serv*, 2004. 55(6): p. 660-4.
[68] Edlin, B. R., et al., Overcoming barriers to prevention, care, and treatment of hepatitis C in illicit drug users. *Clin Infect Dis*, 2005. 40 Suppl 5: p. S276-85.
[69] Treloar, C., J. Rance, and M. Backmund, Understanding barriers to hepatitis C virus care and stigmatization from a social perspective. *Clin Infect Dis*, 2013. 57 Suppl 2: p. S51-5.

[70] Brener, L., et al., Discrimination by health care workers versus discrimination by others: countervailing forces on HCV treatment intentions. *Psychol Health Med,* 2015. 20(2): p. 148-53.

[71] Zevin, B., Managing chronic hepatitis C in primary-care settings: more than antiviral therapy. *Public Health Rep,* 2007. 122 Suppl 2: p. 78-82.

[72] Ti, L., S. Parent, and M. E. Socias, Integrated Models of Care for People Living with Hepatitis C Virus and a Substance Use Disorder: Protocol for a Systematic Review. *JMIR Res Protoc,* 2018. 7(5): p. e122.

[73] Fourati, S., et al., Approaches for simplified HCV diagnostic algorithms. *J Int AIDS Soc,* 2018. 21 Suppl 2: p. e25058.

[74] Harris, K. A., Jr., J. H. Arnsten, and A.H. Litwin, Successful integration of hepatitis C evaluation and treatment services with methadone maintenance. *J Addict Med,* 2010. 4(1): p. 20-6.

In: The Pharmacological Guide to Sofosbuvir   ISBN: 978-1-53616-476-3
Editor: Vijay Gayam   © 2019 Nova Science Publishers, Inc.

Chapter 7

SOFOSBUVIR AND CHRONIC HEPATITIS C TREATMENT FAILURE

Arshpal Gill[1,], MD, Priya Batta[2,†], Amrendra Kumar Mandal[3,‡], MD, Pavani Garlapati[3,§], MD, Vijay Gayam[3,||], MD and Smruti Mohanty[4,#], MD, FACP*
[1]American University of Antigua, Osbourn, Antigua & Barbuda
[2]Windsor University School of Medicine, Basseterre, St.Kitts
[3]Department of Internal Medicine, Interfaith Medical Center, Brooklyn, NY, US
[4]Department of Medicine and Division of Gastroenterology and Hepatology, New York-Presbyterian Brooklyn Methodist Hospital, Brooklyn, NY, US

---

[*] Corresponding Author's E-mail: arshgillmd@gmail.com.
[†] Author's E-mail: Priya.batta@student.windsor.edu.
[‡] Author's E-mail: Amandal@interfaithmedical.com.
[§] Author's E-mail: docpavanireddy@gmail.com.
[||] Author's E-mail: vgayam@interfaithmedical.org.
[#] Author's E-mail: srm9006@nyp.org.

ABSTRACT

Hepatitis C Virus carries a high burden of disease, so the recent development of Direct-Acting Anti-Viral (DAA) is an essential advancement in medical sciences. It replaced the previous less effective interferon-based regimens. When considering a DAA regimen, Sofosbuvir is a vital drug as it is part of a regimen which is successful against all 6 HCV Genotypes, leading to the possibility of a pan-genotypic regimen. While Sofosbuvir and DAA, in general, are both highly effective and well-tolerated treatments, they can still fail. Failure of DAA may be rare, but the consequences of a chronic HCV infection are profound. This chapter discusses factors associated with DAA failure, including Cirrhosis, Vitamin D deficiency, Renal Failure, and Co-Infection with HIV. The impact and role of viral resistance variants in HCV will also be discussed, as well as the management of DAA failure using Sofosbuvir-based regimen.

Keywords: Hepatitis C Virus, direct-acting antivirals, sofosbuvir, treatment failure

1. INTRODUCTION

One of the most prevalent and lethal infections globally is the Hepatitis C Virus. Chronic hepatitis C virus (HCV) is the pre-eminent cause of global mortality due to an infectious agent [1]. HCV may be a life-threatening pathology which can cause both hepatic and extra-hepatic manifestations. As a blood-borne pathogen, it has infected over 185 million people worldwide. If untreated, HCV can result in complications including hepatic cirrhosis, hepatocellular carcinoma (HCC), and ultimately death [2]. The impact of HCV is visible on mortality, as the median age of death in patients with HCV is 53 years, when compared to 81 years, as seen in the general population [3]. Therefore, it is of paramount importance to have a treatment which is successful at eradicating HCV. Successful treatment, defined as Sustained Virologic Response (SVR), can effectively cure HCV, decrease liver scarring and fibrosis, and ultimately decrease the risk of HCC [1]. There are numerous and complex modalities in which

HCV can damage the liver. For instance, inflammasomes can stimulate interleukins and thus lead to inflammation that causes complications such as cirrhosis and HCC [4]. Furthermore, genetic factors called microRNAs can alter liver cirrhosis by converting it into HCC [5].

Sustained Virologic Response (SVR) is the ultimate goal of HCV therapy, as the achievement of SVR will help reduce the overall mortality risk. SVR is defined as undetectable levels of HCV RNA post-treatment [6].

Achieving SVR has been a challenge in the past, as less successful therapies existed, including interferon and ribavirin therapies which will be discussed in this chapter. Fortunately, the advancement of medicine has led to new medications called direct-acting antivirals (DAA) that lead to improved compliance and efficacy [7]. The advent of DAAs has us in an era where treatment is more effective than ever. The gold standard for HCV treatment today is considered to be DAAs as defined by the AASLD guidelines [8].

2. INTERFERON-BASED REGIMENS

The use of interferon and ribavirin had been the previous mainstay treatment for HCV. Interferon-based regimens were very prone to failure. Factors that contributed to a lack of improvement included race, specifically African Americans, and genotype 1 infection [9].

One case study noted that only 19% of patients had an SVR post 24 weeks of interferon treatment [10]. Even a very early double-blind study comparing interferon-based regimens to DAA therapy showed an improved SVR in those with HCV genotype 1, as the interferon group had a response rate of just 40%, while the early DAAs concept showed an SVR of 68%. Also, the DAA regimen was able to reduce treatment duration [11]. Naturally, SVR with DAAs is considerably higher but, it is noteworthy to compare DAAs to interferon in the same trial; which revealed that even in its infancy, DAAs were more potent than interferon-based regimens.

3. RIBAVIRIN

Another treatment option for HCV before DAAs was Ribavirin. Ribavirin has many shortcomings, particularly its side effects. Although its exact mechanism of action is unknown, ribavirin's role in HCV infection before the oral DAA era was to help improve the efficacy of interferon-based regimens, which it was able to do. However, even in the DAA era, Ribavirin may be considered in the right scenario as it has a clinical benefit in specific patient populations [12]. Adverse effects are also a noted problem with Ribavirin. Hemolytic anemia is a dose-dependent side effect, which is both common and morbid [13, 14].

4. DAA FAILURE

Patients treated with interferon and ribavirin had a lower health-related quality of life (HRQOL), and the quality of life was worsened, particularly in those with a higher drop in hemoglobin levels [15]. Not only has the new DAA treatment regimen caused an improved patient experience, but it has also led to increased medication compliance due to higher HRQOL scores [16]. IFN and Ribavirin-free treatment demonstrates an overall high SVR rate of 97.6% [17]. Interferon-based treatments would fail more often as they were not effective concepts in addition to having reduced compliance rates due to its adverse effects. DAA failures are far less common, but there are various topics to address within the realm of DAA failure. Interestingly, the gold standard of DAA failure is another DAA regimen, which will be discussed [8].

4.1. What Causes DAA Failure?

DAAs are an excellent tool at combating HCV. When compared to their predecessors, they demonstrate high efficacy and a much better safety profile. The relative novelty of DAA makes it a challenging topic to assess, as there remains a generalized lack of knowledge in that field. For instance, one large-scale study noted that there was a high failure rate in genotypes 2,3,5 as some patients received an inappropriate regimen [18]. The evolution of DAA guidelines logically will mitigate failures attributed to regimen selection. Furthermore, the creation of a pan-genotypic regimen will reduce errors related to regimen selection. A great example is the Sofosbuvir/Velpatasvir regimen, as it is effective across also genotypes, regardless of prior treatment status or existing cirrhosis and the status of its pan-genotype, is represented in the current AASLD guidelines [8, 19].

4.2. Factors Associated with DAA Failure

DAAs are a relatively novel concept, and as more and more literature develops, clinicians will have a stronger grasp of what may or may not cause DAA failure. It is imperative that clinicians and studies publish their data to see any patterns associated with DAA failure.

It is equally important to remember the role of healthcare workers and communication in the eradication of HCV. Patient perception of treatment will depend on their knowledge along with the information provided to them by the pharmacist. A well-established rapport with the pharmacist, counseling, and education on HCV, adherence to treatment, and access to a pharmacist can alter treatment efficacy [20].

4.3. Existing Cirrhosis in DAA Failure

Cirrhosis is a feared sequela in the natural history of chronic HCV infection. The early stages of HCV infection may be silent, and over the years may develop into fibrosis, which may culminate in cirrhosis [21]. Cirrhosis is a problem as it may interfere with SVR when considering DAA treatment. Fortunately, it appears that there are DAA regimens, which are effective in patients with and without cirrhosis. This can be illustrated in the results of the ASTRAL-1 trial [22], where cirrhosis did not appear to significantly alter both the efficacy and safety of the Sofosbuvir/Velpatasvir regimen.

4.4. Vitamin D Deficiency in DAA Failure

Vitamin D deficiency played a role in various disease processes and was indeed noted to play a role in both interferon failure in HCV infection and to increase the risk of acute liver failure [23]. Vitamin D also appears to play a role in hindering the achievement of SVR with DAAs [24, 25]. Therefore, clinicians should be wary of a potential vitamin D deficiency before initiating DAA therapy.

4.5. HCV/HIV Co-Infection in DAA Failure

HIV used to be a severe problem in interferon-based therapies, but DAAs remains effective even in patients co-infected with HIV/HCV [26]. There are still factors associated with DAA failure in the co-infected population; persons with drug use (PWID), and patients with cirrhosis tend to have a lower SVR when examining the co-infected population [27]. The AASLD recognizes HIV as a potential problem with certain DAAs, as the treatment duration may be extended by 4 weeks in certain sofosbuvir-based regimens if there is indeed a co-infection [8].

4.6. Injection Drug Use

Intravenous drug use can lead to blood-borne diseases, including HIV and HCV. Patients that were co-infected with HCV and HIV that are cirrhotic or IV drug users had a lower SVR response to DAA treatment [27]. Intravenous drug users that develop decompensated cirrhosis or renal insufficiency have increased risk of DAA toxicity and thus, treatment failure [28].

4.7. Renal Failure and DAA Failure

HCV is associated with renal disease, as a significant number of patients will develop renal problems in HCV infection. Furthermore, sofosbuvir is also renally excreted. However, it appears that treatment remains both safe and efficacious with an SVR greater than 90% in most cases [29]. Patients with renal failure may have a harder time achieving SVR12 in DAA therapy. One study noted that patients with a Creatinine Clearance >90 mL/min were less likely to achieve SVR12 when compared to those with a Creatinine Clearance <90mL/min [30]. Based on this data, to achieve optimal results, clinicians should try to treat HCV before renal failure when possible.

5. VIRAL RESISTANCE IN SOFOSBUVIR FAILURE

Viral resistance plays an uncertain role when it comes to HCV and DAA failure. The development of viral resistance-associated substitutions is commonly referred to as RASs.

One large study examined the impact of RASs and DAA therapy. It was noted that RASs might be seen at baseline and develop as a consequence of DAA therapy.

Viral resistance theoretically could achieve SVR a more difficult task, particularly in Sofosbuvir-based regimens. The NS3, Q80K/R NS3, Q80K/R substitution was common in genotype 1a infections, seen 45% of the time, but only 2.6% of the time in genotype 1b infections. RASs at other locations were less common. Interestingly, the baseline NS3 RASs had no impact on achieving SVR12 rates in patients taking Ledipasvir/Sofosbuvir based regimens. One location of significance in genotype 1b infections were baseline polymorphisms at position 316, which were associated with a diminished response rate [31, 32].

Despite all the data on viral resistance, there appears to be a simple solution in achieving SVR in resistance variants; which is to address the treatment duration. Treatment durations less than 98 days demonstrated an SVR of 87%. Treatment durations longer than 98 days showed an SVR of 100%. This is consistent with the thought that longer treatment durations can overcome baselines resistance variants. The effect of increasing treatment duration in viral resistance is noted in the AASLD guidelines [8, 32]. It can be concluded that the practical impact of baseline RAS is uncertain. Clinical studies show that it has little clinical significance when considering DAA therapy, as one study observed that NS5A RAS testing did not enhance outcomes [33]. When considering patients who had baseline RASs and failed DAA therapy, 97% of patients responded to Sofosbuvir/Velpatasvir/ Voxilaprevir; with baselines, RAS being essentially a non-factor in achieving SVR [34]. This likely plays a role in the development of Sofosbuvir/Velpatasvir/Voxilaprevir as an AASLD guideline approved DAA regimen in previous DAA failure [8].

6. SOFOSBUVIR/VELPATASIVR/VOXILAPREVIR AS A SOLUTION TO DAA FAILURE

Sofosbuvir/Velpatasvir/Voxilaprevir represents a triple therapy that is excellent for treating treatment-experienced patients. It demonstrates a consistently high SVR, even in patients with NS5A RASs [35].

Sofosbuvir is an inhibitor of HCV viral replication through its activity as an NS5B inhibitor. It has minimal drug interactions, which makes it an excellent choice to be part of a DAA regimen that consists of at least one other HCV antiviral. Furthermore, renal or hepatic impairment doesn't require dose adjustments with Sofosbuvir [36]. The AASLD guidelines recommend Sofosbuvir in numerous regimens, including the pan-genotypic regimen of Sofosbuvir and Velpatasvir which may be used across all 6 major HCV genotypes [8].

Velpatasvir is an HCV NS5A inhibitor with antiviral activity across HCV viral replicons in all genotypes. The pan-genotypic effects of Velpatasvir are crucial as it may provide clinicians with a DAA regimen in Sofosbuvir/Velpatasvir, which is effective in all genotypes [22, 37]. In addition to Velpatasvirs pan-genotypic activity, it can rapidly reduce HCV RNA levels, which is a part of the reason that the Sofosbuvir/ Velpatasvir/Voxilaprevir combination is an effective re-treatment option in all 6 major HCV genotypes [38].

Voxilaprevir represents an NS3/4A inhibitor that has a strong resistance profile, which makes it effective against RAS. While Sofosbuvir and Velpatasvir is a commonly used regimen in any of the 6 major HCV genotype infections, it is most often considered as an initial DAA regimen. The addition of Voxilaprevir provides clinicians a reliable option in treating DAA failures in HCV across all genotypes [8, 39, 40].

6.1. Sofosbuvir/Velpatasvir/Voxilaprevir for DAA Re-Treatment

The Sofosbuvir/Velpatasvir/Voxilaprevir regimen was thoroughly assessed in the POLARIS-1 and POLARIS-4 landmark clinical trials. The POLARIS-1 and POLARIS-4 assess' patients who have already used a previous DAA regimen. The study population differed based on what type of regimen was given. In POLARIS-1, the patient population included genotype 1 infected patients who previously failed a regimen with an NS5A inhibitor. In POLARIS-4, the patient population included those who did not yet fail an NS5A inhibitor. The Sofosbuvir/Velpatasvir/ Voxilaprevir regimen in POLARIS-1 showed a response rate of 96%. The Sofosbuvir/Velpatasvir/Voxilaprevir regimen showed a response rate of 98% in POLARIS-4. Adverse effects of Sofosbuvir/Velpatasvir/ Voxilaprevir documented in the POLARIS-1 and 4 trials were a headache, fatigue, diarrhea, and nausea. Despite this, serious adverse events were scarce as <1% discontinued therapy due to adverse events [39].

The POLARIS-1 and POLARIS-4 trials success can be illustrated in the current AASLD guidelines for DAA failures, including Sofosbuvir and NS5A failures. The triple-drug regimen of Sofosbuvir/Velpatasvir/Voxilaprevir is an approved Sofosbuvir-based regimen for previous DAA failure, and it is approved for all 6 major HCV genotypes [8].

Conclusion

In summary, clinicians should feel confident in the efficacy and the safety of DAAs, including Sofosbuvir-based regimens in the treatment of HCV. The high success rate, combined with few serious adverse reactions makes DAAs a promising tool when trying to reduce the heavy global burden of disease attributable to HCV. In a small cohort of the population, DAA failure is still possible, with factors including cirrhosis, co-infection with HIV, vitamin D deficiency, patients with a history of drug abuse, and renal failure all having a potentially higher risk of failing DAA therapy. The role of baseline RAS is unclear, but evidence shows that the effect of RAS on SVR appears to be diminutive clinically speaking. Regardless of the cause of failure, Sofosbuvir/Velpatasvir/Voxilaprevir appears to have a high efficacy in patients who have previously failed a DAA regimen.

References

[1] Lledó, G., Benítez-Gutiérrez, L., Arias, A., Requena, S., Cuervas-Mons, V., de Mendoza, C. Benefits of hepatitis C cure with antivirals: why test and treat? *Future microbiology*, 2019; 14(5): 425 - 35.

[2] Venkatesan, A. Review on chemogenomic approaches towards hepatitis C viral targets. *Journal of Cellular Biochemistry*, 2019.

[3] Simmons, R., Ireland, G., Ijaz, S., Ramsay, M., Mandal, S., Borne, NIfHRHPRUiB et al. Causes of death among persons diagnosed with

hepatitis C infection in the pre and post DAA era in England: a record linkage study. *Journal of Viral Hepatitis*, 2019.
[4] Dadmanesh, M., Ranjbar, M. M., Ghorban, K. Inflammasomes and their roles in the pathogenesis of viral hepatitis and their related complications; an updated systematic review. *Immunology Letters,* 2019.
[5] Kanda, T., Goto, T., Hirotsu, Y., Moriyama, M., Omata, M. Molecular Mechanisms Driving Progression of Liver Cirrhosis towards Hepatocellular Carcinoma in Chronic Hepatitis B and C Infections: A Review. *International Journal of Molecular Sciences,* 2019; 20(6):1358.
[6] Swain, M. G., Lai, M. Y., Shiffman, M. L., Cooksley, W. G. E., Zeuzem, S., Dieterich, D. T. et al. A sustained virologic response is durable in patients with chronic hepatitis C treated with peginterferon alfa-2a and ribavirin. *Gastroenterology*, 2010; 139(5):1593 - 601.
[7] FakhriRavari, A., Malakouti, M., Brady, R. Interferon-free treatments for chronic hepatitis C genotype 1 infection. *Journal of Clinical and Translational Hepatology,* 2016;4(2):97.
[8] *AASLD*. https://www.hcvguidelines.org/about.
[9] Shiffman, M. L., Hofmann, C. M., Gabbay, J., Luketic, V. A., Sterling, R. K., Sanyal, A. J. et al. Treatment of chronic hepatitis C in patients who failed interferon monotherapy: effects of higher doses of interferon and ribavirin combination therapy. *The American Journal of Gastroenterology,* 2000; 95(10):2928.
[10] Poynard, T., Marcellin, P., Lee, S. S., Niederau, C., Minuk, G. S., Ideo, G. et al. Randomised trial of interferon α2b plus ribavirin for 48 weeks or 24 weeks versus interferon α2b plus placebo for 48 weeks for treatment of chronic infection with hepatitis C virus. *The Lancet,* 1998; 352(9138):1426 - 32.
[11] Poordad, F., McCone, Jr. J., Bacon, B. R., Bruno, S., Manns, M. P., Sulkowski, M. S. et al. Boceprevir for untreated chronic HCV genotype 1 infection. *New England Journal of Medicine,* 2011; 364(13):1195 - 206.

[12] Feld, J. J., Jacobson, I. M., Sulkowski, M. S., Poordad, F., Tatsch, F., Pawlotsky, J. M. Ribavirin revisited in the era of direct-acting antiviral therapy for hepatitis C virus infection. *Liver International,* 2017; 37(1):5 - 18.

[13] Sato, S., Moriya, K., Furukawa, M., Saikawa, S., Namisaki, T., Kitade, M. et al. Efficacy of L-carnitine on ribavirin-induced hemolytic anemia in patients with hepatitis C virus infection. *Clinical and Molecular Hepatology,* 2019.

[14] Soota, K., Maliakkal, B. Ribavirin-induced hemolysis: a novel mechanism of action against chronic hepatitis C virus infection. *World Journal of Gastroenterology: WJG,* 2014; 20(43):16184.

[15] Malik, A., Kumar, K., Malet, P., Ostapowicz, G., Adams, G., Wood, M. et al. A randomized trial of high-dose interferon alpha-2b, with or without ribavirin, in chronic hepatitis C patients who have not responded to standard dose interferon. *Alimentary Pharmacology and Therapeutics,* 2002; 16(3):381 - 8.

[16] Hollander, A., Foster, G. R., Weiland, O. Health-related quality of life before, during and after combination therapy with interferon and ribavirin in unselected Swedish patients with chronic hepatitis C. *Scandinavian Journal of Gastroenterology,* 2006; 41(5):577 - 85.

[17] Cacoub, P., Bourliere, M., Asselah, T., De Ledinghen, V., Mathurin, P., Hézode, C. et al. French Patients with Hepatitis C Treated with Direct-Acting Antiviral Combinations: The Effect on Patient-Reported Outcomes. *Value in Health,* 2018; 21(10):1218 - 25.

[18] Kondili, L. A., Gaeta, G. B., Brunetto, M. R., Di Leo, A., Iannone, A., Santantonio, T. A., et al. Incidence of DAA failure and the clinical impact of retreatment in real-life patients treated in the advanced stage of liver disease: Interim evaluations from the PITER network. *PloS One,* 2017; 12(10):e0185728.

[19] Mir, F., Kahveci, A. S., Ibdah, J. A., Tahan, V. Sofosbuvir/ velpatasvir regimen promises an effective pan-genotypic hepatitis C virus cure. *Drug Design, Development and Therapy,* 2017; 11:497.

[20] Gomes, L. O., Teixeira, M. R., da Rosa, J. A., Foppa, A. A., Rover, M. R. M., Farias, M. R. The benefits of a public pharmacist service in

chronic hepattis C treatment: The real-life results of sofosbuvir-based therapy. *Research in Social and Administrative Pharmacy*, 2019.
[21] Seeff, L. B. The history of the "natural history" of hepatitis C (1968 - 2009). *Liver International*, 2009; 29:89 - 99.
[22] Feld, J. J., Jacobson, I. M., Hézode, C., Asselah, T., Ruane, P. J., Gruener, N. et al. Sofosbuvir and velpatasvir for HCV genotype 1, 2, 4, 5, and 6 infection. *New England Journal of Medicine,* 2015; 373(27):2599 - 607.
[23] García-Álvarez, M., Pineda-Tenor, D., Jiménez-Sousa, M. A., Fernández-Rodríguez, A., Guzmán-Fulgencio, M., Resino, S. Relationship of vitamin D status with advanced liver fibrosis and response to hepatitis C virus therapy: a meta-analysis. *Hepatology,* 2014; 60(5):1541 - 50.
[24] Kondo, Y. Hepatitis C infected patients need vitamin D3 supplementation in the era of direct acting antivirals treatment. *World Journal of Gastroenterology*, 2017; 23(8):1325.
[25] Gayam, V., Mandal, A. K., Khalid, M., Mukhtar, O., Gill, A., Garlapati, P. et al. Association Between Vitamin D Levels and Treatment Response to Direct-Acting Antivirals in Chronic Hepatitis C: A Real-World Study. *Gastroenterology Research*, 2018; 11(4): 309.
[26] Collins, L. F., Chan, A., Zheng, J., Chow, S.-C., Wilder, J. M., Muir, A. J. et al., editors. Direct-acting antivirals improve access to care and cure for patients with HIV and chronic HCV infection. *Open Forum Infectious Diseases,* 2017: Oxford University Press US.
[27] Rossi, C., Young, J., Martel-Laferrière, V., Walmsley, S., Cooper, C., Wong, A. et al., editors. Direct-Acting Antiviral Treatment Failure Among Hepatitis C and HIV–Coinfected Patients in Clinical Care. *Open Forum Infectious Diseases*, 2019: Oxford University Press US.
[28] Soriano, V., Labarga, P., de Mendoza, C., Fernández-Montero, J. V., Esposito, I., Benítez-Gutiérrez, L. et al. New hepatitis C therapies for special patient populations. *Expert Opinion on Pharmacotherapy,* 2016; 17(2):217 - 29.

[29] Lens, S., Rodriguez-Tajes, S., Llovet, L.-P., Maduell, F., Londoño, M.-C. Treating hepatitis C in patients with renal failure. *Digestive Diseases,* 2017; 35(4):339 - 46.

[30] Jansen, J. W., Powderly, G. M., Linneman, T. W. Identification of predictors for treatment failure in hepatitis C virus patients treated with ledipasvir and sofosbuvir. *Annals of Pharmacotherapy,* 2017; 51(7):543 - 7.

[31] Donaldson, E. F., Harrington, P. R., O'Rear, J. J., Naeger, L. K. Clinical evidence and bioinformatics characterization of potential hepatitis C virus resistance pathways for sofosbuvir. *Hepatology,* 2015; 61(1):56 - 65.

[32] Wang, G. P., Terrault, N., Reeves, J. D., Liu, L., Li, E., Zhao, L. et al. Prevalence and impact of baseline resistance-associated substitutions on the efficacy of ledipasvir/sofosbuvir or simeprevir/sofosbuvir against GT1 HCV infection. *Scientific Reports,* 2018; 8(1):3199.

[33] Real, L. M., Macías, J., Pérez, A. B., Merino, D., Granados, R., Morano, L. et al. Baseline resistance-guided therapy does not enhance the response to interferon-free treatment of HCV infection in real life. *Scientific Reports,* 2018;8.

[34] Sarrazin, C., Cooper, C. L., Manns, M. P., Reddy, K. R., Kowdley, K. V., Roberts, S. K. et al. No impact of resistance-associated substitutions on the efficacy of sofosbuvir, velpatasvir, and voxilaprevir for 12 weeks in HCV DAA-experienced patients. *Journal of Hepatology,* 2018; 69(6):1221 - 30.

[35] Bourlière, M., Pietri, O., Castellani, P., Oules, V., Adhoute, X. Sofosbuvir, velpatasvir and voxilaprevir: a new triple combination for hepatitis C virus treatment. One pill fits all? Is it the end of the road? *Therapeutic Advances in Gastroenterology,* 2018; 11: 1756284818812358.

[36] Cuenca-Lopez, F., Rivero, A., Rivero-Juárez, A. Pharmacokinetics and pharmacodynamics of sofosbuvir and ledipasvir for the treatment of hepatitis C. *Expert Opinion on Drug Metabolism and Toxicology,* 2017; 13(1):105 - 12.

[37] Foster, G. R., Afdhal, N., Roberts, S. K., Bräu, N., Gane, E. J., Pianko, S. et al. Sofosbuvir and velpatasvir for HCV genotype 2 and 3 infection. *New England Journal of Medicine*, 2015; 373(27): 2608 - 17.

[38] Lawitz, E., Freilich, B., Link, J., German, P., Mo, H., Han, L. et al. A phase 1, randomized, dose-ranging study of GS-5816, a once-daily NS 5A inhibitor, in patients with genotype 1–4 hepatitis C virus. *Journal of Viral Hepatitis*, 2015; 22(12):1011 - 9.

[39] Bourlière, M., Gordon, S. C., Flamm, S. L., Cooper, C. L., Ramji, A., Tong, M. et al. Sofosbuvir, velpatasvir, and voxilaprevir for previously treated HCV infection. *New England Journal of Medicine*, 2017; 376(22):2134 - 46.

[40] Rodriguez-Torres, M., Glass, S., Hill, J., Freilich, B., Hassman, D., Di Bisceglie, A. et al. GS-9857 in patients with chronic hepatitis C virus genotype 1–4 infection: a randomized, double-blind, dose-ranging phase 1 study. *Journal of Viral Hepatitis*, 2016; 23(8): 614 - 22.

EDITOR'S CONTACT INFORMATION

Dr. Vijay Gayam
Assistant Program Director, Dept. of Medicine, Interfaith Medical Center;
Clinical Assistant Professor of Medicine,
SUNY Downstate University Hospital;
Adjuct Professor of Medicine, American University of Antigua;
Councilor, Eastern section, American Federation for Medical Research
E-mail: vgayam@interfaithmedical.org

INDEX

#

7.4. HCV Genotype 4, 50

A

access, 92, 126, 151, 161
acid, 27, 40, 158
acid-reducing medications, 27
acute hepatitis, 3
acute infection, 42, 60, 62
adjustment, 12, 13, 26, 27, 28, 104
adverse effects, 2, 13, 14, 15, 16, 19, 40, 48, 71, 137, 152, 153, 174, 179
adverse event, 15, 16, 22, 41, 47, 48, 69, 70, 71, 92, 97, 98, 99, 103, 114, 117, 134, 136, 145
Africa, 17, 36, 72
age, 3, 14, 16, 30, 43, 52, 62, 82, 106, 111, 127
ALT, 21, 22, 114, 124
American Association for the Study of Liver Diseases- Infectious Disease Society of America (AASLD-IDSA), 43, 46, 49, 53, 96, 98, 100, 102, 103, 104, 107, 108, 137, 138, 146, 150, 158, 161, 165
amiodarone, 14, 23, 24, 31, 37, 38
anemia, 16, 19, 45, 61, 63, 92, 117, 140, 141, 143, 152
antiretrovirals, 26, 38, 130
antiviral agents, 3, 37, 107, 114
antiviral therapy, 32, 34, 38, 41, 42, 54, 95, 97, 111, 125
ART, 114, 115, 117, 118, 121, 122, 126
assessment, 43, 107, 126, 127
asthenia, 103, 152, 153
atazanavir, 26, 118, 119, 120, 122, 123, 124, 129

B

baby boomers, 3
barriers, 64, 117, 159, 160, 161
BCRP, 2, 24, 25, 31, 123, 124
BCRP/ABCG2 related drugs, 24
benefits, 44, 67, 139
bilirubin, 19, 20, 123
blood, 3, 6, 42, 60, 61, 73, 117, 160
bradycardia, 23, 31, 143

C

calcineurin inhibitors, 27, 104

carcinoma, 70, 107, 151
CDC, 3, 31, 135, 158
chemotherapy, 21, 33, 57
children, 14, 15, 30, 34, 111
Child-Turcotte-Pugh (CTP), 7, 92, 93, 96, 97, 98, 99, 100, 101
chronic hepatitis, v, vi, vii, viii, 3, 34, 35, 37, 39, 40, 41, 46, 54, 55, 56, 57, 59, 82, 86, 87, 88, 94, 102, 108, 129, 130, 131, 134, 135, 167, 168, 181, 183
chronic hepatitis C, v, vi, vii, 32, 34, 35, 36, 37, 38, 39, 40, 41, 42, 52, 53, 54, 55, 56, 57, 59, 82, 83, 84, 86, 87, 88, 92, 102, 108, 110, 111, 114, 127, 128, 129, 130, 131, 132, 134, 135, 164, 167, 168, 169, 181, 182, 183, 185
chronic kidney disease (CKD), 94, 107, 110, 121, 130
CKD, 13, 93, 94, 102
cleavage, 7, 11, 30
clinical trials, 14, 26, 40, 45, 46, 47, 52, 53, 64, 97, 101, 115, 116, 117, 122, 126
combination therapy, 8, 14, 16, 18, 25, 26, 27, 29, 106
community, 47, 48, 50, 54, 56, 71, 72, 73, 74, 108, 131, 160
comorbidity, viii, 134, 158
compensated cirrhosis, 49, 60, 62, 65, 66, 71, 72, 74, 75, 76, 77, 78, 79, 81, 94, 95, 100, 103, 116, 119, 122, 150, 152, 154
complications, viii, 2, 41, 93, 101, 113, 125, 129, 138, 158
contraindications, 2, 19
corticosteroids, 105
cost, 2, 16, 62, 64, 67, 68, 82, 92, 105
counseling, 158, 159, 160
cure, 2, 4, 6, 18, 27, 71, 72
cyclosporine, 104, 105
CYP 3A4 inducers, 26
cytochrome, 64, 111, 119

D

DAA failure, viii, 148, 149, 150, 172, 174, 175, 176, 177, 178, 179, 180, 182
daclatasvir, 7, 16, 17, 18, 24, 29, 32, 34, 47, 48, 49, 56, 65, 75, 76, 77, 89, 93, 96, 98, 99, 100, 101, 103, 109, 115, 118, 119, 128, 129, 135, 139, 145, 146, 165
daclatasvir plus sofosbuvir, 56, 115, 118, 165
darunavir, 26, 118, 119, 120, 122, 124
deaths, 98, 141, 143, 151
decompensated cirrhosis, 12, 17, 30, 33, 34, 60, 66, 74, 75, 80, 81, 85, 89, 93, 94, 95, 96, 97, 98, 99, 100, 101, 105, 109, 127, 148, 149, 150, 151, 176
decompensated liver cirrhosis, vii, 92, 95
detectable, 4, 21, 22, 42, 117, 125, 138
detection, 32, 111, 124, 158
dialysis, 13, 30, 94, 102
diarrhea, 71, 144, 145, 157
direct-acting antiviral agents, 114
direct-acting antivirals, 17, 20, 35, 38, 39, 40, 41, 56, 57, 60, 63, 83, 86, 89, 92, 107, 108, 114, 115, 128, 129, 130, 134, 135, 136, 164, 165, 167, 172, 173, 183
direct-acting anti-virals, 60
disease progression, 4, 74, 117
diseases, 2, 35, 53, 57, 107, 108, 110, 115, 135, 158
disorder, 136, 159, 160, 161
distribution, 25, 31, 82, 85, 162
DNA, 20, 21, 22, 124, 125
dolutegravir, 26, 118, 120, 122, 130
dosage, 13, 22, 119
dosing, 2, 13, 27, 41
dosing regimens, 2
drug interaction, vii, 2, 16, 23, 24, 25, 27, 31, 38, 64, 92, 105, 106, 111, 114, 115, 117, 118, 119, 121, 123, 124, 126, 129, 130

Index

drug-drug interactions, vii, 2, 64, 92, 105, 106, 114, 117, 119, 124, 128, 130
drugs, vii, viii, 2, 5, 6, 7, 8, 17, 24, 25, 26, 27, 28, 30, 32, 34, 35, 36, 53, 81, 82, 119, 120, 122, 134, 135, 137, 153, 157

E

education, 43, 159, 160
efavirenz, 25, 26, 118, 119, 120, 122, 123, 128, 129
elbasvir, 7, 24, 38, 77, 150, 156
end-stage renal disease, 34, 94, 107
enzyme, 2, 4, 7, 8, 11, 20, 24, 26, 31, 64, 74, 105, 119, 122, 123, 124
ESRD, 13, 30, 93, 94, 102
everolimus, 105
evidence, 13, 20, 38, 51, 102, 106, 159, 161
exclusion, 74, 153, 155
exposure, 10, 21, 23, 27, 64, 73, 116, 130

F

fibrosis, viii, 16, 41, 43, 44, 50, 54, 57, 61, 62, 68, 74, 85, 114, 115, 127, 137, 141
fidelity, 8, 31, 63
filtration, 11, 12, 30, 92, 102, 121
flaviviridae family, 2, 3
food, 11, 27, 44
Food and Drug Administration (FDA), 4, 13, 14, 15, 16, 20, 21, 31, 34, 35, 37, 40, 41, 45, 46, 50, 51, 63, 93, 99, 111, 135, 138, 154, 156
France, 97, 153, 162

G

generalizability, 152, 153, 157
genome, 5, 36, 64

genotype, 2, 4, 14, 15, 17, 18, 29, 32, 33, 34, 36, 41, 45, 46, 47, 48, 49, 50, 51, 52, 53, 54, 55, 56, 57, 63, 65, 66, 67, 72, 73, 75, 83, 85, 86, 87, 88, 94, 95, 96, 97, 98, 99, 100, 101, 103, 106, 108, 109, 110, 111, 116, 118, 119, 120, 121, 122, 125, 128, 131,143, 144, 152
genotype 2 and 3 HCV infections, 18
geriatrics, 2, 15, 19
glecaprevir/pibrentasvir, 115, 128
guidance, 36, 85, 123, 131, 161
guidelines, 29, 32, 35, 68, 70, 73, 75, 115, 118, 121, 124, 131, 137, 138

H

half-life, 10, 11, 23, 64
HBV, vi, viii, 3, 15, 20, 21, 22, 37, 93, 102, 113, 114, 124, 125, 126, 131
HBV infection, 20, 21, 114, 125, 126
HCC, 40, 41, 42, 44, 92, 93, 104, 105, 106, 111
HCV Genotype 1, 45, 83, 84, 85, 166
HCV Genotype 2, 48, 83, 166
HCV Genotype 3, 49, 70
HCV genotypes, 2, 17, 30, 35, 37, 44, 47, 51, 52, 62, 63, 65, 69, 72, 103, 172, 179, 180
headache, 14, 15, 19, 45, 47, 48, 67, 69, 103, 139, 140, 141, 142, 143, 144, 152, 153, 155, 157
health, 16, 44, 65, 72, 106, 135, 137, 151, 158, 159, 160, 161
health care, 44, 65, 72
hemodialysis, 23, 34, 110
hepatic fibrosis, 41, 54, 61, 74
hepatic impairment, 12, 99, 178
hepatitis, vii, 2, 3, 13, 17, 18, 20, 21, 31, 32, 33, 34, 35, 36, 37, 38, 39, 40, 42, 43, 51, 52, 53, 54, 55, 56, 57, 82, 83, 84, 85, 86, 87, 88, 92, 94, 106, 107, 108, 109, 110,

111, 113, 114, 115, 117, 125, 127, 128, 129, 130, 131, 132, 134, 135, 145, 158, 160, 161, 162
hepatitis B, viii, 3, 20, 21, 37, 43, 93, 102, 113, 114, 125, 131, 160, 163
hepatitis B virus, 43, 114, 131
hepatitis B Virus, 37, 93
hepatitis C, vi, vii, viii, 2, 3, 4, 9, 13, 15, 17, 18, 23, 31, 32, 33, 34, 35, 36, 37, 38, 39, 40, 42, 43, 46, 51, 52, 53, 54, 55, 56, 57, 60, 61, 65, 66, 82, 83, 84, 85, 86, 87, 88, 89, 92, 93, 94, 106, 107, 108, 109, 110, 111, 113, 114, 115, 117, 127, 128, 129, 130, 131, 133, 134, 135, 145, 146, 150, 157, 158, 161, 162, 163, 164, 165, 166, 167, 168, 169, 171, 172, 180, 181, 182, 183, 184, 185
hepatocellular carcinoma, 2, 3, 41, 52, 54, 60, 61, 62, 69, 92, 93, 107, 118, 125, 134, 151
hepatocellular carcinoma (HCC), 2, 3, 40, 41, 42, 44, 52, 54, 60, 61, 62, 69, 92, 93, 104, 105, 106, 107, 111, 118, 125, 134, 151, 172, 181
hepatorenal syndrome, 92
high-risk populations, 134, 138, 158, 162
history, 7, 32, 53, 60, 62, 67, 83, 105, 127, 131, 134, 136, 137, 159
HIV related drugs, 25
HIV/HCV co-infected, 115, 139, 140, 141, 142
HIV-1, 56, 89, 128
human, 23, 56, 108, 114, 115, 129
human immunodeficiency virus (HIV), vi, viii, 3, 12, 17, 19, 25, 26, 38, 40, 43, 46, 47, 48, 56, 73, 74, 88, 89, 93, 94, 108, 113, 114, 115, 116, 117, 118, 120, 121, 122, 123, 124, 126, 127, 128, 129, 130, 139, 140, 141, 142, 146, 147, 151, 152, 158, 160

I

identification, 33, 138, 162
IFN, 6, 19, 37, 40, 41, 44, 48, 51, 76, 77, 131, 134, 136, 154, 156, 162
illicit drug use, 3, 153, 158
immunodeficiency, viii, 56, 108, 113, 114, 115, 129
incidence, 16, 45, 61, 62, 94, 127, 135
individuals, viii, 2, 12, 15, 17, 20, 21, 22, 62, 64, 66, 70, 73, 74, 92, 115, 127, 128, 132, 134, 138, 151, 158, 159, 162
infection, vii, viii, 2, 3, 4, 14, 16, 17, 18, 19, 20, 21, 31, 33, 34, 35, 36, 38, 41, 42, 43, 44, 45, 46, 47, 48, 49, 51, 52, 53, 54, 55, 56, 57, 60, 61, 63, 65, 67, 68, 69, 70, 71, 72, 73, 74, 75, 82, 84, 85, 86, 88, 92, 94, 96, 98, 99, 100, 102, 106, 108, 109, 110, 111, 113, 115, 116, 117, 118, 120, 121, 124, 126, 127, 128, 129, 130, 131, 134, 135, 138, 139, 141, 143, 146, 153, 155, 158, 159, 161, 162
inhibition, 7, 24, 33, 138
inhibitor, 7, 8, 10, 18, 26, 30, 31, 32, 33, 39, 41, 46, 53, 57, 65, 105, 109, 111, 115, 122, 129, 138, 139, 144, 147, 148, 149, 150, 154, 156
injection drug use (IDU), 134, 136, 137, 145, 151, 155, 158, 164, 176
insomnia, 19, 45, 67, 142, 144, 152, 155
interferon, 2, 15, 16, 20, 36, 40, 41, 46, 54, 55, 57, 60, 61, 63, 72, 74, 81, 87, 88, 99, 116, 117, 125, 129, 131, 134, 136, 152
interferon and ribavirin, 2, 4, 15, 61, 63, 84, 87, 88, 125, 163, 173, 174, 181, 182
interferon-based regimens, 60, 61, 63, 74, 81, 99, 172, 173, 174
International Network on Hepatitis in Substance Users (INHSU), 135, 137
intervention, 62, 94, 159, 160

Index

L

ledipasvir, 7, 13, 14, 15, 16, 17, 18, 26, 28, 29, 33, 34, 37, 45, 46, 50, 51, 55, 56, 57, 65, 66, 67, 68, 71, 73, 76, 77, 78, 80, 83, 84, 85, 86, 88, 93, 96, 100, 102, 103, 106, 108, 110, 115, 118, 119, 120, 121, 128, 129, 130, 135, 145, 146, 152, 166, 167, 177, 184

ledipasvir/sofosbuvir, 26, 29, 45, 50, 51, 65, 66, 67, 68, 71, 73, 85, 96, 100, 108, 115, 119, 120, 121, 146, 167, 177, 184

liver, vii, viii, 2, 3, 6, 7, 14, 18, 20, 21, 32, 33, 34, 39, 41, 42, 43, 44, 48, 51, 53, 54, 56, 57, 60, 62, 74, 85, 92, 93, 94, 95, 96, 98, 99, 100, 104, 106, 107, 108, 109, 110, 111, 114, 115, 118, 124, 125, 127, 129, 140, 141, 146, 147, 148, 149, 150, 151, 158

liver cirrhosis, vii, 42, 48, 92

liver disease, viii, 3, 6, 7, 14, 32, 33, 39, 42, 43, 44, 51, 57, 62, 74, 92, 93, 96, 106, 108, 114, 115, 127, 141, 151

liver failure, 2, 20, 33, 98, 125

liver transplant, 2, 3, 18, 33, 34, 42, 43, 48, 56, 60, 62, 92, 94, 100, 107, 108, 109, 111, 127, 140, 146, 147, 148, 149, 150

liver transplantation, 2, 3, 33, 34, 42, 43, 48, 56, 60, 62, 83, 92, 93, 100, 107, 109, 110

lopinavir, 26, 118, 119, 122

M

majority, 45, 61, 97, 99, 103, 125

management, vii, viii, 17, 22, 43, 53, 88, 106, 107, 115, 121, 125, 130, 134, 138, 159, 160, 161

mechanism of action, 2, 5, 9, 64, 174, 182

medical, vii, 92, 95, 106, 108, 158

MELD score, 92, 95, 98

mental illness, viii, 134, 136, 137, 138, 151, 154, 156, 157, 158, 160, 161, 162, 163, 168

meta-analysis, 21, 37, 52, 54, 94, 102, 110, 115, 127, 136

metabolized, 10, 30, 74, 123, 138

morbidity, viii, 2, 40, 48, 113, 115, 117

mortality, viii, 2, 6, 40, 42, 44, 52, 54, 62, 75, 94, 101, 102, 111, 113, 115, 117, 129

mortality rate, 40, 62, 101

mycophenolate mofetil, 105

N

nausea, 14, 19, 45, 47, 48, 67, 71, 139, 140, 141, 142, 143, 144, 145, 152, 155, 157

nevirapine, 25, 26, 118, 119

New England, 33, 35, 37, 55, 56, 109, 110

North America, 103, 136, 158

NS2, 5

NS3, 2, 5, 7, 8, 17, 28, 30, 64, 77, 84, 115, 130, 137, 138, 147, 148, 149, 150, 154, 156, 177, 179

NS3/4A protease inhibitors, 2, 7, 8, 17, 30, 138

NS4A, 5

NS4B, 5

NS5 B, 5

NS5A, 2, 5, 7, 8, 17, 18, 28, 29, 30, 32, 40, 46, 57, 64, 65, 78, 79, 94, 96, 111, 115, 122, 129, 138, 139, 144, 145, 148, 149, 150, 152, 154, 156, 166, 178, 179, 180

NS5A failures, 149, 150, 180

NS5A inhibitors, 2, 7, 8, 17, 29, 30, 32, 40, 46, 64, 94, 138, 145, 150, 156

NS5B inhibitors, 2, 7, 8

NS5B polymerase, vii, 2, 4, 7, 8, 17, 30, 31, 33, 39, 40, 53, 64, 115

nucleoside inhibitor, 7, 33, 39

Index

O

ombitasvir, 7, 109, 128, 131
opioid substitution therapy (OST), 135, 137, 153, 155, 164, 167
organ, 3, 25, 115, 122, 151

P

participants, 15, 46, 116, 120, 122, 155, 159
pathology, 61, 62, 82
pathway, 11, 28, 38, 45
pediatrics, 2, 14, 19
Persons Who Inject Drugs (PWID), 134, 136, 151, 153, 155, 158, 161, 176
P-glycoprotein, 2, 24, 25
pharmacokinetics, 2, 10, 11, 12, 14, 30, 33, 34, 84, 110, 111, 184
pharmacology, vii, 32, 82
phosphorylation, 8, 11, 28, 30
placebo, 22, 46, 50, 143, 154, 157
policymakers, 60, 61, 63, 82
polymerase, vii, 2, 4, 7, 8, 9, 17, 30, 31, 32, 33, 39, 40, 41, 53, 60, 63, 115, 138
population, 2, 12, 13, 19, 30, 38, 47, 50, 62, 68, 69, 72, 73, 85, 102, 105, 115, 116, 117, 134, 135, 138, 139, 151, 157, 158, 160
post-liver transplantation, 48, 56, 99, 165
post-transplantation, 17, 92
pregnancy, 13, 14, 94, 106, 111
pregnancy and breastfeeding, 13
prevention, 52, 92, 99, 131, 136, 138, 158
protease inhibitors, 2, 8, 17, 30, 41, 122, 127, 138, 139, 149, 150
psychiatrist, 126, 159, 160
public health, 60, 61, 63, 82, 114, 134, 136, 137, 138, 159

R

race, 47, 52, 68, 87
raltegravir, 26, 118, 120, 122, 128
RAS, 29, 76, 148
real-world data, 101, 151
recommendations, iv, 17, 32, 85, 94, 101, 102, 127, 134, 137, 138, 161
recurrence, 34, 56, 62, 98, 101, 109
regression, 54, 116, 117
renal impairment, vii, 12, 30, 92, 102, 106
renal transplant, 103, 107
replication, vii, 2, 5, 6, 7, 8, 20, 21, 30, 63, 64, 84, 94, 115, 125, 129, 138, 139
resistance, viii, 2, 8, 24, 28, 29, 31, 32, 38, 41, 43, 45, 56, 64, 69, 84, 135, 152, 172, 177, 178, 179, 184
resistance-associated variants, 152
resources, 67, 126, 160
response, 3, 4, 6, 16, 27, 32, 41, 48, 52, 54, 62, 63, 64, 66, 70, 72, 73, 75, 87, 92, 93, 108, 114, 116, 117, 122, 123, 128, 129, 131, 134, 137, 139, 151, 156, 162
rilpivirine, 26, 118, 120, 122, 128
risk, 2, 3, 13, 14, 16, 20, 21, 22, 24, 41, 62, 68, 69, 74, 86, 94, 102, 106, 107, 110, 111, 114, 120, 121, 124, 125, 126, 135, 136, 158, 159, 160, 161
risk factors, 41, 68, 107
RNA, 3, 5, 6, 7, 9, 17, 29, 30, 40, 41, 42, 46, 63, 64, 71, 84, 85, 117, 119, 120, 125, 138, 147, 152, 158

S

safety, vii, 13, 14, 16, 24, 30, 32, 34, 40, 41, 47, 48, 49, 50, 52, 53, 67, 69, 70, 86, 94, 95, 98, 101, 104, 106, 109, 110, 119, 121, 122, 123, 124, 131, 134, 136, 138, 139, 151, 153, 154, 155, 162
secretion, 11, 12, 25, 30

Index

serum, 20, 42, 51, 57, 122, 125
services, iv, 126, 158, 159, 160, 161, 162
showing, 64, 71, 156
side effects, 2, 4, 6, 18, 19, 36, 60, 61, 63, 67, 136
signs, 23, 44, 68
simeprevir /sofosbuvir, 121
six hepatitis, 18
sofosbuvir and daclatasvir combination, 139
sofosbuvir/velpatasivr/voxilaprevir, 178
sofosbuvir/velpatasvir, 25, 26, 27, 29, 46, 49, 50, 51, 65, 66, 67, 68, 69, 70, 71, 72, 73, 75, 97, 98, 101, 122, 123, 124, 148, 149, 156, 167, 175, 176, 178, 179, 180
state, 23, 74, 137
substance abuse, 73, 116, 136, 161
substance use, 134, 137, 138, 157, 159, 160, 161, 162
substance use disorders, vi, viii, 133, 134, 157, 159, 161, 162, 165
substitution, 28, 29, 137
substitutions, 8, 28, 29, 151
substrate, 10, 24, 25, 26, 30, 64, 105, 123, 124
suppression, 21, 71, 94, 115, 125
survival, 52, 89, 92, 106
sustained virological response (SVR12), 4, 6, 16, 22, 41, 45, 47, 49, 51, 54, 66, 74, 86, 87, 95, 98, 99, 101, 103, 104, 116, 117, 118, 119, 120, 122, 151, 152, 153, 154, 155, 157, 162, 177
symptoms, 23, 42, 44, 61, 136, 151
syndrome, 92, 95, 121
synthesis, 7, 9, 10

T

tacrolimus, 27, 104, 105
target, 6, 7, 70, 105, 111, 115, 160
testing, 29, 63, 76, 85, 124, 127, 134, 158, 160

therapy, 2, 4, 6, 15, 16, 17, 18, 20, 21, 22, 23, 26, 27, 28, 29, 30, 35, 39, 42, 43, 46, 47, 51, 57, 62, 64, 65, 68, 75, 81, 83, 88, 93, 94, 96, 97, 101, 104, 107, 111, 114, 115, 117, 119, 120, 121, 122, 123, 124, 125, 126, 127, 128, 132, 135, 136, 137, 138, 140, 141, 142, 143, 144, 145, 153, 155
toxicity, 27, 119, 120, 121, 124
transmission, viii, 3, 29, 44, 53, 73, 94, 108, 113, 126, 136, 159
transplant, 2, 19, 43, 48, 62, 94, 99, 103, 104, 107, 110, 111, 139, 140, 146, 147, 148, 149, 150
transplant recipients, 2, 94, 103, 104, 107, 110, 111
transplantation, 21, 62, 83, 92, 93, 95, 99, 109, 110, 122, 140
treatment failure, vi, 18, 32, 61, 96, 117, 139, 154, 171, 172, 177, 183, 184
treatment naïve, 17, 47, 48, 49, 80, 81, 119, 139, 140, 141, 142, 143, 144, 145, 147, 148, 149, 152, 153, 154
trial, 14, 22, 33, 35, 36, 46, 47, 48, 50, 51, 55, 57, 65, 66, 67, 68, 70, 72, 73, 88, 96, 97, 98, 99, 101, 103, 106, 111, 118, 119, 121, 128, 131, 139, 140, 141, 142, 143, 144, 145, 152, 153, 155, 157

U

upper respiratory tract, 141, 143, 153
urine, 12, 30, 45, 137

V

velpatasvir, 7, 13, 17, 18, 27, 33, 36, 46, 49, 50, 51, 55, 56, 65, 66, 69, 70, 72, 75, 76, 77, 78, 79, 80, 81, 83, 84, 85, 86, 92, 94, 96, 100, 102, 104, 109, 111, 115, 118, 123, 124, 129, 130, 135, 145, 148, 154,

164, 166, 167, 178, 179, 182, 183, 184, 185
virus infection, 20, 32, 33, 34, 35, 36, 38, 52, 53, 54, 56, 82, 83, 86, 92, 106, 107, 109, 110, 111, 127, 134, 162
viruses, viii, 60, 113
vitamin d levels, 51, 57, 183
vomiting, 71
voxilaprevir, 7, 18, 26, 46, 49, 50, 55, 66, 70, 76, 77, 78, 79, 80, 84, 102, 104, 118, 123, 124, 130, 135, 145, 148, 149, 154, 156, 164, 166, 167, 178, 179, 180, 184, 185

W

warfarin, 26, 38
World Health Organization (WHO), 4, 31, 40, 135, 137, 162
worldwide, 39, 92, 115, 135

Pharmaceutical Innovation: Challenges and Competitors

Editors: Tomas E. Sanchez and Charles L. Scott

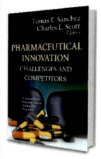

Series: Pharmacology - Research, Safety Testing and Regulation

Book Description: This book examines the challenges associated with striking the proper balance between lower cost drugs and maintaining an innovative domestic pharmaceutical sector.

Hardcover ISBN: 978-1-62257-068-3
Retail Price: $130

Human Serum Albumin (HSA): Functional Structure, Synthesis and Therapeutic Uses

Editor: Travis Stokes

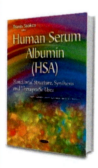

Series: Protein Biochemistry, Synthesis, Structure and Cellular Functions

Book Description: This book provides an overview of the expanding field of preclinical and clinical applications and developments that use albumin as a carrier of drug delivery systems.

Hardcover ISBN: 978-1-63482-963-2
Retail Price: $230

Antibiotic Resistance: Causes and Risk Factors, Mechanisms and Alternatives

Editors: Adriel R. Bonilla and Kaden P. Muniz

Series: Pharmacology - Research, Safety Testing and Regulation

Book Description: This book addresses the concern that over the past few years, there has been a major rise in resistance to antibiotics among gram-negative bacteria. New antibacterial drugs with novel modes of actions are urgently required in order to fight against infection.

Hardcover ISBN: 978-1-60741-623-4
Retail Price: $265

Medicinal Plants and Sustainable Development

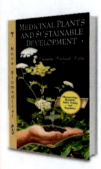

Editor: Chandra Prakash Kala (Indian Institute of Forest Management, Madhya Pradesh, India)

Series: Pharmacology - Research, Safety Testing and Regulation

Book Description: This book deals with multidisciplinary approach and contains information on different aspects of medicinal plants, which can be used as guiding tools.

Hardcover ISBN: 978-1-61761-942-7
Retail Price: $139